# Living with Parkinson's Disease

# Living with Parkinson's Disease

**Kathleen E. Biziere, M.D., Ph.D.**
Senior Technical Advisor
Quintiles, BRI, Inc.
Alexandria, VA

*AND*

**Matthias C. Kurth, M.D., Ph.D.**
Assistant Clinical Director
Barrow Neurological Institute
Phoenix, Arizona

## demos vermande ◆

**Demos Vermande, 386 Park Avenue South, New York, New York 10016**

**Library of Congress Cataloging-in-Publication Data**

Bizière, K.
  Living with Parkinson's disease / Kathleen E. Biziere and Matthias
Kurth
    p.    cm.
  Includes index.
  ISBN 1-888799-10-2
  1. Parkinsonism—Popular works.    I. Kurth, Matthias.    II. Title.
RC382.B54    1996
616.8'33   dc21                                          95 16622
                                                         CIP

Made in the United States of America

*This book is dedicated to Bob, the brave young man who taught us how much patients need to understand research on their disease, and with how much hope they wait for the cure.*

# CONTENTS

# PREFACE

Parkinson's disease is one of the most common neurologic disorders, affecting many people over the age of 40 and more than 15 percent of all people over age 65. This book is written specifically for anyone who has been diagnosed with Parkinson's disease, their family members and friends, and for physicians and other health care providers who help to manage the disease. It will serve as a guide to learning about the disease and its potential impact on your life. It describes the nature of Parkinson's disease and treatments that are available for its management, as well as the results of research efforts devoted to the discovery of improved treatments. This is a time of great excitement in research and rapid advances in clinical management, such that most people diagnosed with the disease can continue to lead full and productive lives.

Parkinson's disease is due to the gradual loss of a small group of nerve cells located deep within the brain in an area called by its Latin name, the *substantia nigra*. The symptoms of the disease result from decreased concentrations of dopamine, a substance normally produced by the lost cells. Its treatment focuses on the replacement of this missing dopamine. This works well during the early stages of the disease, but replacing dopamine does not prevent the slow loss of substantia nigra nerve cells from continuing, and therapy becomes increasingly less satisfactory over time. Although the ultimate goal of research is the discovery of a cure that will prevent the continuing inexorable loss of nerve cells in the substantia nigra, current research is also focused on the development of treatments that allow patients to maintain a good response even during the later stages of the disease.

Section I discusses the symptoms and brain lesions that characterize Parkinson's disease, the management of its primary symptoms with levodopa, the management of secondary symptoms and complications, surgical treatments, and the concept of "wellness" in living with chronic illness.

Section II reviews research devoted to improving the management of the disease, including the development of treatments that will prolong the effectiveness of levodopa, the search for longer acting agents, and the improvement of late-stage complications of the disease. This is followed by chapters that discuss the search for a cure for the disease and prospects for replacing the neurons lost as a result of the disease process. Of particular interest is a detailed discussion of clinical trials, their role in the development of new therapies, and points to be considered before participating.

Our hope is that this book will enable everyone affected by Parkinson's disease to better understand its nature and treatment, make current research efforts understandable, and provide evidence that there is room for reasonable optimism. Our dream is that this book will soon become obsolete because the cure for Parkinson's disease will have been discovered.

# Section

# I

# THE DISEASE AND ITS MANAGEMENT

# 1

# What Is Parkinson's Disease?

Depictions that suggest the symptoms of Parkinson's disease can be found in ancient Egyptian hieroglyphs that go back more than 4,000 years. The Greeks, Romans, and perhaps even the Bible mention conditions that can best be described as parkinsonism. Yet it was not until 1817 that this mysterious disorder of the nervous system achieved a distinctive and memorable description that has stood the test of time. In a short and succinct treatise entitled "On the Shaking Palsy," James Parkinson presented in simple terms the hallmarks of this disabling disorder that involved:

> ". . . involuntary tremulous motion, with lessened muscular power, in parts not in action and even when supported; with a propensity to bend the trunk forward, and to pass from a walking to a running pace: the senses and intellect being uninjured."

What is this disorder that intrigues thousands of physicians and researchers in the hope of understanding the deep inner workings of the brain and hope of soon finding a cure?

The simplest definition of Parkinson's disease is based on the clinical features that characterize those affected by it—the presence of at least two of the following—trembling, slowness of movement, and stiffness of muscles. To these hallmarks, known as the classic "parkinsonian triad," must be added

3

a tendency to stand in a stooped position, to walk with short shuffling steps, and to speak softly in a rapid even tone.

The cause of the disease remains unknown, and no definitive diagnostic test allows a physician to say with certainty that a person has Parkinson's disease. The clinical history and neurologic examination are the best diagnostic tools available. It is therefore not surprising that the final diagnostic accuracy remains at best 80–90 percent, even in the most experienced centers dedicated to the treatment of Parkinson's disease. The 10–20 percent of patients initially misdiagnosed as suffering from the disease are often subsequently diagnosed as having other diseases of the brain that resemble Parkinson's disease.

Precise information concerning the number of people who have Parkinson's disease is limited, but it is usually estimated that it affects approximately one million people in the United States. One recent study estimated that as many as 15 percent of those aged 65 to 74 years and 29 percent of those aged 75 to 84 have symptoms of Parkinson's disease. Alzheimer's disease is found in up to 40 percent of all individuals over the age of 65, totaling between 3 million and 6 million Americans. Heart disease afflicts more than 50 million, cancer more than 5 million, and diabetes approximately 12 million. Thus, it is not surprising that Parkinson's disease, although common, is often not the first diagnosis considered by well-trained and astute clinicians faced with patients who have mild and often less than classic symptoms. Some people may never be diagnosed, while others eventually make their own diagnosis through reading and discussion with numerous health care providers.

## ▶ PRIMARY SYMPTOMS

Parkinson's disease rarely affects people under the age of 40, and its average age of onset is about 60. The onset of Parkinson's disease is very gradual, and the first signs of the disease often appear long before the person is aware of them. Especially if the first sign is not one of the classic triad of tremor, rigidity, and bradykinesia, the correct diagnosis may not be made for many years. The average time from initial onset of symptoms to diagnosis is estimated to be from two to four years.

In order to make the diagnosis of Parkinson's disease, the physician must eliminate other possibilities, such as a tumor or stroke. The most important component of this process of "differential diagnosis" is an accurate medical history, followed by a physical examination. The physician may also need to order tests such as a CAT scan or a magnetic resonance imaging (MRI) scan, and may do blood tests as well.

The first signs of the disease, such as postural changes or stiffness of a limb, may be noticed by others. The person may notice changes that seem to be vague and nonspecific, such as a lack of energy, tiredness, or difficulty in accomplishing tasks that once were simple.

Trembling or tremor is most often the first symptom that appears, often on one side of the body and often only as small movements of an arm or leg. It tends to occur in the affected limbs at rest and to disappear during movement and sleep. This distinguishes it from the tremor seen in other diseases and explains why it is called a *resting tremor*. It often is worsened by nervousness or intense concentration. A condition called *micrographia* is often present, in which the handwriting becomes small and tends to become even smaller as the person continues to write.

Most people recall the presence of tremor for many months before they decided to seek medical attention. They typically consult their physician because other symptoms of Parkinson's disease have impaired their function or because the extent of their tremor is sufficient to interfere with everyday activities.

Some patients have little or no tremor in the early stage of the disease, with rigidity and bradykinesia being the first symptoms seen. This may manifest itself as a sense of "weakness" in an arm or leg. In many cases the first symptoms are seen primarily on one side of the body.

The most troubling symptom of Parkinson's disease is slowness of bodily movements, or "bradykinesia" (from the Greek *brady* meaning slow and *kinesia* meaning movement). This problem contributes significantly to the disabilities reported by patients, including difficulties in getting out of chairs and cars and turning over in bed, trouble performing fine motor tasks such as buttoning clothing, and slowness in walking. People with bradykinesia have difficulty doing two things at the same time or switching quickly from one activity to another. They also have difficulty initiating new movements. Many people with Parkinson's disease find that their balance is impaired. Early in the course of the disease this is most often not a true balance problem, but rather due to slowness in initiating the correct moves to catch themselves when they start to fall.

Another common complaint is a sense of "weakness" and an inability to perform tasks that seem to require only strength—such as opening a jar or using a can opener. When carefully analyzed, these tasks actually require coordination more than strength, and it is the inability to *coordinate* a number of muscles correctly that is actually responsible for these complaints. Again, the underlying reason is bradykinesia, not true muscle weakness.

Another manifestation of bradykinesia is the loss of automatic movements such as swinging the arms during walking, eye blinking, swallowing saliva, and expressive movements of the face and hands. All these often unconscious movements are absent in those with severe bradykinesia. Reduced eye blinking gives a staring expression to the face and can cause irritation of the eyes. Decreased swallowing of saliva causes drooling. An often surprising characteristic of bradykinesia is its variability—patients can do things on one occasion but not another. Family members and friends sometimes find these sudden changes confusing.

Rigidity is the third classic symptom of Parkinson's disease. It is the component of the parkinsonian triad that is most often not initially noticed by the patient, but rather is detected by the examining physician. This symptom translates into resistance to passive movements around the joints. Physicians usually look for it around the elbow joint. In Parkinson's disease, movement is jerky, as if there were a cogged wheel in the joint. Rigidity is often overlooked by patients early in the illness. As Parkinson's disease progresses, people may become acutely aware of stiffness at the end of each dose of medication. Rigidity may be perceived as a sense of "stiffness," but also as tiredness, aching, or soreness. When this happens, rigidity becomes one of the symptoms that interferes significantly with quality of life.

## ▶ SECONDARY SYMPTOMS

The hallmarks of tremor, slowness of movements, and stiffness of muscles are not the only symptoms of Parkinson's disease, or even the most disabling. Many people report a reduction in their handwriting size months to years before other motor symptoms affect quality of life. Others relate that their family members noticed a change in their facial expression suggestive of being depressed or "more withdrawn," before other symptoms were perceived. Long before neurologic signs and symptoms are noted, up to 15 percent of people with Parkinson's disease may have experienced at least one episode of severe depression, sometimes accompanied by anxiety, preceding other symptoms of PD.

People with Parkinson's disease may experience symptoms that affect their walking and balance; affect swallowing, digestion, and elimination; alter their sleep patterns; and produce a number of other symptoms that may be more irritating than disabling. These symptoms are discussed in detail in Chapter 3.

## ▶ BRAIN LESIONS THAT UNDERLIE THE SYMPTOMS OF PARKINSON'S DISEASE

Although James Parkinson described the clinical features of Parkinson's disease in 1817, their physical cause was not understood until the 1960s.

As early as the 1920s, researchers studying the brains of patients with Parkinson's disease described the loss of a group of nerve cells deep within the brain in an area called the *substantia nigra*. These cells contain a dark pigment called *melanin*; hence the name of the brain region in which they are found (in Latin *nigra* means black). Loss of substantia nigra nerve cells is one of the hallmarks of Parkinson's disease. Another characteristic was that substantia nigra nerve cells found in the process of dying contained pink iridescent inclusions, called *Lewy bodies* after their discoverer. At the beginning of the twentieth century, however, little was known about the function of these big, darkly pigmented cells of the substantia nigra or their Lewy body inclusions. A possible relationship between the loss of this small group of nerve cells and the symptoms of Parkinson's disease was therefore largely overlooked until the advent of modern neurochemistry in the early 1960s.

By the end of the 1950s, scientists learned that nerve cells use simple chemical substances called *neurotransmitters* to communicate with one another. The early 1960s saw a blossoming of techniques to identify and measure neurotransmitters in the brain, and new ones were discovered at a rapid pace. *Dopamine* was identified as an important neurotransmitter that seemed to be involved in a number of brain functions. Researchers observed that in Parkinson's disease the concentrations of this simple chemical was diminished in a particular brain region called the *corpus striatum*. This clue eventually led to an understanding of the relationship between the mysterious loss of substantia nigra pigmented cells and the symptoms of Parkinson's disease. Advances in techniques for the identification of neurotransmitters in neurons then led to the discovery that dopamine is made by the large pigmented neurons of the substantia nigra.

Scientists showed that these neurons send long projections called axons to a brain region located about an inch away, the *corpus striatum* (Figure 1.1). Dopamine is made in the cell body of substantia nigra nerve cells and stored in the terminal part of the axons. Thus, the connection between the two abnormalities that characterized Parkinson's disease became obvious, namely the loss of substantia nigra nerve cells and decreased concentrations of dopamine in the striatum. At this point our current understanding of the disease took shape.

Today we know that substantia nigra nerve cells make dopamine and release it from their terminals in the striatum. Parkinson's disease is due to the progressive loss of these nerve cells, gradually leading to a profound decrease in concentrations of dopamine in the striatum. This in turn causes the symptoms of Parkinson's disease. The concentration of dopamine in the striatum must be decreased by approximately 80 percent or more for symptoms of Parkinson's disease to first appear.

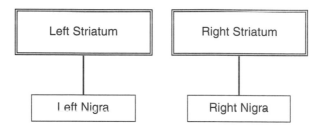

*Figure 1.1* Schematic representation of the connections between the substantia nigra and the corpus striatum. Nerve cells located in the substantia nigra send long projections called axons to the striatum. These cells make dopamine and store it in the terminal part of their axons, then release it as needed. In Parkinson's disease the nerve cells in the substantia nigra are slowly lost. As a consequence the levels of dopamine in the striatum gradually decrease.

## ►BIOCHEMISTRY OF PARKINSON'S DISEASE

How does dopamine exert its effects in the striatum? Normally, dopamine is continually released from its storage sites into the synaptic cleft, a narrow space that separates two nerve cells. On the other side of the synaptic cleft, striatal neurons carry "receptors" to which dopamine binds (Figure 1.2).

The interaction of dopamine with its receptors turns on a cascade of events that leads to dopamine's effects. In a certain sense, the interaction of dopamine with its receptors is similar to the interaction of a key with a lock; a key fits its lock, and this allows a door to open. The symptoms of Parkinson's disease are due to decreased stimulation of dopamine receptors.

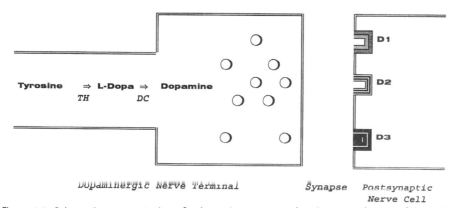

*Figure 1.2* Schematic representation of a dopamine synapse, showing several types of dopamine receptors. Dopamine is made in dopaminergic nerve terminals and stored in small vesicles. D1, D2, and D3 receptors are not usually found together on the same postsynaptic cell.

Understanding the biochemistry of Parkinson's disease led to treatments that replaced the missing dopamine. Since the symptoms of Parkinson's disease appeared to be due to decreased concentrations of dopamine in the corpus striatum, scientists reasoned that one way to overcome the symptoms would be to treat patients with dopamine. However, this substance cannot enter the brain and has significant side effects. Investigators therefore decided to give patients a substance that could enter the brain and be transformed there into dopamine. This substance was *levodopa*. The use of high dose levodopa in the mid-1960s led to the modern era of medical therapy of Parkinson's disease. Levodopa is the active ingredient of Sinemet® and Madopar® (not available commercially in the United States). No better treatment has yet been discovered. Chapter 2 reviews the mechanism of action of levodopa and related medications, their side effects, and their use in the treatment of Parkinson's disease. Many new approaches for the treatment of Parkinson's disease are currently being researched and tested throughout the world; they are described in Section II.

## ►CONDITIONS OFTEN MISTAKEN FOR PARKINSON'S DISEASE

### Essential Tremor

Many people subsequently diagnosed with Parkinson's disease are initially diagnosed with *essential tremor*, a common condition that affects up to 3 million Americans. Conversely, people who actually have this relatively benign condition often fear that they have Parkinson's disease, especially if someone close to them has the disease. Up to half of all individuals affected by essential tremor report a strong family history of the disorder, and the condition is then called *familial tremor*. Essential tremor is clinically different from the tremor found in Parkinson's disease. First, there are *no* additional neurologic findings except for the tremor, i.e., no stiffness or slowness. Second, the tremor is absent at rest and is only noted with action and posture of a limb. Third, the tremor is less likely to be asymmetric and more likely to involve the head and voice. Patients may have a tremulous voice and a "no" or "yes" head nodding tremor. Medication for essential tremor may help control tremor in patients with Parkinson's disease, but antiparkinsonian medications do not help people with essential tremor.

### Drug-Induced Parkinsonism

Medications commonly used for a number of medical conditions can cause parkinsonism. Fortunately, the parkinsonian symptoms usually fade away within a few weeks after the responsible medication is withdrawn.

Drugs that cause parkinsonism share the common property of preventing the action of dopamine in the striatum. The main group of Parkinson-producing drugs are the *neuroleptics*, or major tranquilizers, used in the treatment of mental illnesses called *psychoses*, especially the psychosis found in schizophrenia.

Agents used in the treatment of nausea and other stomach problems often block the effects of dopamine. These medications are frequently prescribed to elderly people and are often an unsuspected cause of parkinsonism.

A few antihypertensive agents (drugs that treat elevated blood pressure) may cause parkinsonism because they deplete dopamine from the brain by destroying the storage vesicles in the nerve terminals. These medications are rarely prescribed now because of their ability to induce both parkinsonism and severe depression in some subjects.

### Atypical Parkinsonism

Not everyone who presents with slowness, stiffness, and tremor has typical (also called *idiopathic*) Parkinson's disease. About 20 percent of those who at first appear to have Parkinson's disease eventually develop signs and symptoms of a group of disorders classified as "atypical parkinsonism," also called *parkinson plus*, because they have parkinsonian symptoms plus others that are due to loss of nerve cells in other brain areas, such as the cerebellum. Because more than one set of nerve cells is lost, these diseases are also called *multiple system atrophy*. Unfortunately, they respond less well to treatments that help patients with idiopathic Parkinson's disease.

### Progressive Supranuclear Palsy

The most common of the parkinson plus disorders is progressive supranuclear palsy or PSP. It is easily mistaken for Parkinson's disease during its initial course, but after two to three years patients develop severe difficulty with eye movements, which points to the correct diagnosis. The eyes appear fixed in the face and a sense of anguish seems to dominate the expression of patients with PSP. Another feature that distinguishes PSP from Parkinson's disease is the early presence of balance problems (postural instability). Some patients complain of falling long before any other parkinsonian symptom can be detected. Later in the course of PSP patients may develop *retrocollis*, a tendency for the neck to bend back and up, instead of the more typical forward stooped posture of idiopathic Parkinson's disease.

PSP progresses significantly more rapidly than idiopathic Parkinson's disease. Perhaps most disabling is the relative lack of benefit patients receive from medications. Patients are usually run through the gamut of antiparkinsonian medications without significant benefit before the actual diagnosis is made. No effective therapy is known.

### Striatonigral Degeneration

The symptoms of *striatonigral degeneration* are very similar to those of Parkinson's disease, but the disease is characterized by a reduced response to antiparkinsonian medications. Other differentiating features include a tendency for patients to experience *dystonia* (painful sustained muscle contractions) early in the illness, even before starting levodopa therapy. Voice changes, breathing problems, and autonomic nervous system dysfunction (i.e., problems with blood pressure, sweating, and sexual function) tend to be observed sooner than with typical Parkinson's disease. Most patients have some response to antiparkinsonian medications early in the course of the disease, but later develop complications such as an increased likelihood to experience dystonia with each dose of medication. The course is somewhat slower than PSP, but faster than Parkinson's disease.

### Shy-Drager Syndrome

This disease is characterized by "autonomic insufficiency" (problems with blood pressure, sweating, and sexual function), combined with symptoms of cerebellar and basal ganglia dysfunction. Most patients first develop autonomic insufficiency, including orthostatic hypotension (sudden and profound decreases in blood pressure when changing from sitting to standing position that can lead to fainting), impaired sweating, and impotence. Parkinsonian features develop later and include slowness of movement, stiffness, and impaired balance; or cerebellar features such as a wide-based gait, incoordination, and action tremors. As the disease progresses, urinary and rectal incontinence, as well as vocal cord paralysis leading to hoarseness, may occur. Occasional patients may need a tracheotomy or selective botulism toxin injections to relieve severe *stridor* (difficulty breathing) due to to vocal cord paralysis. Treatment is difficult and revolves around management of orthostatic hypotension with agents that increase blood pressure. While levodopa is helpful for the parkinsonian features, it may significantly exacerbate orthostatic hypotension.

### Olivopontocerebellar Atrophy (OPCA)

OPCA is the term used to describe a heterogeneous group of rare neurodegenerative conditions that involve loss of nerve cells in two brain areas, namely the *pons* and the *cerebellum*. Loss of nerve cells in the substantia nigra is also a frequent feature. These syndromes are now also called *spinocerebellar atrophy* (SCA), since selective degeneration of nerve cells in the spinal cord is often associated with pons and cerebellar lesions. Both sporadic and inherited forms are known. At least three genes that lead to this disorder have been identified. No effective therapies are known.

## ▶ NEURODEGENERATIVE DISORDERS: A UNIFYING CONCEPT

Parkinson's disease and atypical parkinsonism belong to a wider group of diseases called *neurodegenerative disorders* that affect the brain and spinal cord. They include conditions such as Alzheimer's disease, Huntington's disease, amyotrophic lateral sclerosis (ALS; Lou Gehrig's disease). All are due to the gradual loss of certain sets of nerve cells in specific areas of the brain. For example, in Huntington's disease a group of neurons located in the *corpus striatum* gradually degenerate. In Alzheimer's disease, several neuronal systems degenerate, including a group of neurons located at the base of the brain. In Lou Gehrig's disease, small groups of neurons in the cerebral cortex, brain stem, and spinal cord gradually disappear. What causes nerve cells to gradually die in these diseases is still unknown, but is the subject of intense research because discovering the cause might lead to a cure. Some researchers believe that some causes may be common to several of these diseases, thus increasing the chances of finding a cure.

## ▶ CONCLUSION

Parkinson's disease is a complex neurodegenerative condition that affects more than one million Americans. Its manifestations and symptoms can affect people in many unique ways. No specific test exists at this time to diagnose the condition with 100 percent certainty. Diagnosis must be made by an experienced physician. Many conditions can mimic Parkinson's disease, as can the use of some commonly used medications. It is not surprising that the diagnosis of Parkinson's disease is at best correct in 80–90 percent of cases. Nevertheless, correct diagnosis is the first step in proper treatment and justifies consultation with experts in this area of neurology.

Although Parkinson's disease cannot be "cured," successful treatments are available that permit people with the disease to live with it successfully. As discussed in Section II of this book, ongoing research holds the promise of future treatments that will manage the symptoms of the disease more successfully and that offer the possibility of slowing or stopping its progress.

# 2

# Managing the Disease Process

The symptoms of Parkinson's disease are the direct result of the loss of dopamine-producing cells from the substantia nigra, as discussed in Chapter 1. All modern management of Parkinson's disease involves replacement of this missing dopamine. Dopamine itself is prevented from entering the brain by a complex mechanism called the blood-brain barrier. Instead, therapy makes use of a precursor of dopamine that does pass this blood-brain barrier and is transformed into dopamine within the brain. High dose levodopa therapy began in the late 1960s and revolutionized the treatment of patients with Parkinson's disease. It is still unquestionably the best treatment for Parkinson's disease and will most probably continue to be the mainstay of therapy until the cause of Parkinson's disease is known and treatment is available to halt the disease process.

Unfortunately, levodopa has numerous side effects, resulting in complications that have occupied the attention of researchers for the last 20 years. Adjunctive medications have helped to reduce side effects and add significantly to the available options for the treatment of Parkinson's disease. Hope now exists that some of these agents may reduce progression of the disease by interfering with the disease process itself, rather than simply treating its symptoms.

## ►DRUGS CURRENTLY USED TO TREAT THE SYMPTOMS OF PARKINSON'S DISEASE: SINEMET® AND MADOPAR®*

Levodopa is the active ingredient of Sinemet® and Madopar®. When taken by mouth, levodopa passes through the stomach, is absorbed from the small bowel, enters the bloodstream, and eventually reaches the brain. A number of factors can affect its absorption from the bowel. For example, the presence of food in the stomach can significantly delay the entrance of levodopa into the bowel. Chemically, levodopa is a large neutral amino acid. Certain proteins, notably those found in meat, liberate neutral amino acids in the stomach and gut during digestion, where they "compete" with levodopa for absorption into the bloodstream. The net result of this competition is that less levodopa is absorbed. This is why Sinemet® and Madopar® do not work as well if they are taken after a large meal, particularly one that contains a lot of meat. Additional difficulties need to be overcome after it has passed into the bowel. For example, factors that decrease gastric emptying can significantly slow the absorption of levodopa and delay the onset of its therapeutic effect.

Once absorbed into the bloodstream, levodopa travels throughout the body and most of it is rapidly eliminated. Only half survives in the bloodstream after 90 minutes (levodopa therefore is said to have a plasma "half-life" of 90 minutes). A small amount of levodopa enters the brain and is taken up by the remaining substantia nigra nerve cells. Within these cells, it is converted to dopamine and stored in small vesicles located in their terminals. Dopamine is continuously released from these vesicles into the striatum at a relatively steady rate as needed.

This storage and slow release of dopamine by nerve cells is why the effect of levodopa initially lasts several hours, despite its rapid clearance from the bloodstream. The gradual release of dopamine from nerve endings is responsible for the smooth, complication-free response to levodopa seen in patients with early mild parkinsonism. However, as the number of substantia nigra nerve cells continues to decline, the amount of dopamine that can be stored in the remaining nerve vesicles becomes increasingly limited. The smooth effects of levodopa observed in early-stage patients then give way to motor fluctuations.

---

* Madopar is not available in the United States.

## ►LEVODOPA IS ADMINISTERED WITH DECARBOXYLASE INHIBITORS

Inside nerve cells, levodopa is converted into dopamine by an enzyme called a decarboxylase (DC) (see Figure 2.1). Because this enzyme is also present in the blood vessels, dopamine is formed in the bloodstream and produces side effects such as nausea, vomiting, and decreased blood pressure.

Carbidopa and benserazide block DC but do not penetrate the brain. They are used to prevent the conversion of levodopa to dopamine in the bloodstream, thus minimizing side effects at the same time that they allow conversion to take place in the brain. Levodopa is normally given in combination with one of these drugs. Sinemet® is the combination of levodopa and carbidopa; Madopar® is the combination of levodopa and benserazide. This combination of DC inhibitors with levodopa markedly reduces side effects and has tremendously improved the quality of life of people with Parkinson's disease.

The dose of DC inhibitor may vary. At least 75 mg per day of carbidopa is needed to effectively block DC, but some people may require up to 150 mg per day. This is easily achieved using a combination of different Sinemet® preparations. While not demonstrated in a rigorous manner, most investigators agree that doses of carbidopa higher than 350 mg per day may cross the blood-brain barrier and interfere with the production of dopamine in the brain. Therefore, the recommended dose of carbidopa is 75–200 mg per day in three or four divided doses.

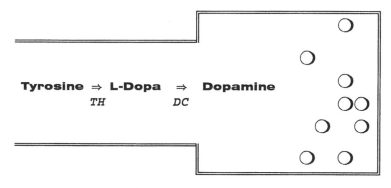

**Tyrosine** ⇒ **L-Dopa** ⇒ **Dopamine**
     *TH*                *DC*

**Dopaminergic Nerve Terminal**

*Figure 2.1.* Nerve cells make dopamine from tyrosine and from levodopa. Two enzymes are needed in this process: TH (tyrosine hydroxylase) and DC (decarboxylase).

## ▶RESPONSE TO LEVODOPA

A good response to levodopa is usual for some years after diagnosis, but it tends to become less helpful with time. This occurs because complications develop rather than because levodopa loses its efficacy. For example, about 50 percent of all patients develop significant motor complications such as dyskinesias and end-of-dose deterioration after about five years of chronic levodopa therapy. The mechanisms that lead to these problems and their potential treatment have become a major focus of research and are discussed in Chapter 10.

When motor fluctuations begin, patients start to feel the effect of each dose of levodopa—they can tell when it begins to work and when its effect wears off (end-of-dose deterioration). They also begin to experience some return of parkinsonian symptoms in the morning before they take their first daily dose. The effect of each dose of levodopa no longer lasts long enough, probably because of a decreasing number of substantia nigra nerve cells to store dopamine. Additionally, new symptoms that do not respond well to levodopa make their appearance as Parkinson's disease progresses. These can include speech and gait disturbances, postural instability (problems with balance), and freezing episodes (during which people find their feet and legs completely immobilized or "frozen" to the ground).

## ▶SIDE EFFECTS OF LEVODOPA

### Nausea and Vomiting

Despite the use of DC inhibitors, levodopa therapy still causes nausea and vomiting in some people. Dopamine stimulates the area postrema, or "vomiting center" located at the junction of the brain and the spinal cord. This area "senses" when something poisonous or dangerous is present in the blood and causes vomiting to prevent further intoxication. Nerve cells in this center use dopamine as their neurotransmitter and are activated by drugs that increase the concentrations of dopamine or stimulate dopamine receptors. Fortunately, the DC inhibitors associated with levodopa are partially taken up by the vomiting center and prevent to some degree the formation of dopamine in this region. This is why a substantial reduction in the number of people plagued by nausea and vomiting occurs with Sinemet® and Madopar® as compared to levodopa alone.

Some patients continue to have this unpleasant side effect even with Sinemet® and Madopar®, especially at the start of treatment. Within three to six months, the vomiting center usually develops tolerance to the increase in dopamine concentrations and no longer reacts. Women tend to be more sensitive than men, although the reason for this is unknown. Unfortunately, the dose of levodopa that causes nausea and vomiting is practically the same as that which improves motor function. Decreasing the dose of levodopa to avoid nausea and vomiting is therefore not helpful. A number of "tricks" can help minimize this side effect. Since the vomiting center becomes accustomed to levodopa, it can be helpful to begin treatment with a low dose and increase it slowly. The vomiting center is particularly sensitive to rapid increases in dopamine concentrations in the bloodstream. Taking levodopa with a meal slows its absorption and thus decreases the likelihood of developing nausea. Finally, caffeine increases the effects of dopamine on this center, so it may be prudent to avoid caffeine during the first weeks of treatment.

### Involuntary Movements

Many people with Parkinson's disease develop abnormal involuntary movements after some years of therapy. These "dyskinesias" include twitches, jerks, and twisting or writhing movements, or they may be limited to simple restlessness. These movements can be just as uncomfortable and disabling as the parkinsonian symptoms. If they occur when medication reaches maximal blood levels after each dose, they are referred to as "peak-dose dyskinesias." Some patients develop involuntary movements at the beginning or end of a dose of medication, called complex dyskinesias.

### Mental Symptoms

Dopamine has an activating effect on the cerebral cortex, and people often report feeling more alert and energetic when they begin treatment with levodopa. The energizing effects of levodopa may cause insomnia and can even lead to feelings of nervousness, inner tension, and jitteriness when they are pronounced. These effects usually subside after a few weeks of treatment; if they do not, they can be controlled with minor tranquilizers such as the benzodiazepines. Levodopa may also cause vivid dreams. Normally this is not a problem, but it may occasionally be distressing and cause nightmares. This effect of levodopa also tends to wane with time. If it persists, a simple way to deal with the problem is to eliminate or decrease the bedtime dose.

Increased sexual interest has been described as a side effect of levodopa. Most people do not experience much change in libido, and those who do usually see it as a return to normal.

Levodopa can cause confusion in a small number of patients, including visual hallucinations and irrational behavior. A rare side effect is mania, characterized by hyperactivity and feelings of grandiosity. Patients start having too many activities and rather ambitious plans, and they sleep less and less. Drugs that block confusion and mania act by blocking a specific dopamine receptor in the brain, but they cannot be used in patients with Parkinson's disease because they also block the beneficial effects of levodopa on parkinsonian symptoms. These "mental" side effects are therefore difficult to treat. They require that all other medications be stopped if possible and that the dose of levodopa be cautiously decreased and adjusted to what the person can tolerate.

Clozapine® is a drug used primarily for the treatment of schizophrenia. It blocks mainly a specific dopamine receptor called D4. Unlike D2 receptor blockers, Clozapine® does not cause parkinsonism. Clinical trials have shown that Clozapine® blocks confusion and hallucinations in patients with Parkinson's disease without worsening their parkinsonian symptoms. However, this drug has a number of unpleasant side effects and can induce the problem of agranulocytosis, in which white blood cells are lost and fatal infectious diseases can develop. White blood cells return to normal two to three weeks after withdrawing Clozapine®, but patients are at high risk during that period. Approximately one percent of patients on Clozapine® develop this complication, and it is mandatory that white blood cell counts be checked weekly.

Ondansetron®, a drug that blocks serotonin receptors, was recently shown in a small study to improve mental symptoms, without suppressing the antiparkinson effect of levodopa. Thus, Ondansetron® might be a safer alternative to Clozapine®. Further studies are needed to confirm the finding.

## ►IMPROVING LEVODOPA THERAPY

One of the problems with regular Sinemet® or Madopar® tablets is the short half-life of levodopa in the bloodstream and the consequent need for frequent dosing throughout the day. Blood and brain levels peak within 30 to 60 minutes after dosing, and then rapidly decrease over the following three to four hours. In early-stage patients these "ups and downs" in levodopa concentrations are a source of discomfort but not a serious problem. Patients in the early stages of Parkinson's disease store dopamine in their substantia nigra nerve cells and release it as needed, which helps to smooth out the oscillations of levodopa in the bloodstream. During the later stages of the disease, few nerve cells are left in the substantia nigra and storage is no longer possible. As a result, the response to therapy begins to oscillate with the levels of levodopa in the bloodstream. Some late-stage patients feel that they spend their days "swinging on" and "swinging off" medication. When they swing on they have side effects due to high concentrations of levodopa; when they swing off, then motor function is poor.

In addition to its short half-life, levodopa induces variable responses from one dose to another. This is a real problem for many people, who feel they can never quite trust their medication. This unpredictable nature of the response to levodopa appears to be at least partly due to variations in gastrointestinal function that in turn lead to erratic absorption. In early stages of Parkinson's disease these issues are more of a nuisance than anything else. In late-stage disease, however, patients become extremely sensitive to even small changes in blood levodopa levels because of increasing neuronal loss. At this stage of the disease, regular absorption of levodopa from the bowel becomes critical.

Swinging on and off and unpredictable response are not seen when levodopa is infused intravenously, confirming that these motor fluctuations are linked to oscillating levels of levodopa in the bloodstream.

### Controlled-Release Formulations of Levodopa

For many years, researchers have looked for ways to obtain improved and prolonged gastrointestinal uptake of levodopa in the hope that this would lead to more sustained blood levels. One method is to make Sinemet® or Madopar® tablets that release levodopa in the stomach and in the bowel over a period of several hours, which avoids abrupt increases and decreases in levodopa brain levels. Encased in a special matrix, the Sinemet CR® tablet dissolves slowly in the stomach and bowel, allowing for a prolonged, steady absorption of levodopa into the bloodstream. Madopar HBS® (not available in the United States) is a capsule that releases levodopa slowly in the stomach (HBS stands for hydrodynamically balanced system). Both seem to be effective in reducing end-of-dose wearing-off.

Many people with Parkinson's disease report a reduction in "off" time and fewer motor fluctuations with the controlled release forms of levodopa. Another advantage of these preparations is that fewer doses per day are needed for symptom control. On the whole, patients often prefer controlled release preparations because of the smoother effect and longer duration of action. Those who experience end-of-dose wearing-off are most likely to benefit from them. However, the controlled release preparations usually take longer than normal tablets to take effect. This is particularly inconvenient with the first morning dose, but can be successfully overcome by taking standard levodopa at that time. Unfortunately, delayed gastric emptying, competition with other neutral amino acids present in digesting proteins, and other interfering effects can limit the benefit of controlled release preparations just as is the case of immediate-release preparations.

Recent research described in Chapter 10 suggests that some late-stage complications such as end-of-dose wearing-off and dyskinesias are related to subtle brain damage due to the sudden rises and falls in brain levodopa levels. If this is true, the occurrence of these complications might be delayed by using the controlled release preparation in the early stages of the disease, long before the onset of motor complications. Many investigators are now of the opinion that the use of controlled release preparations should not be reserved for late-stage patients and insist that these preparations may increase quality of life at all stages of the disease. A double-blind, controlled clinical trial is ongoing with Sinemet CR® to examine whether this is true.

### Drinkable Solutions of Levodopa/Carbidopa

Levodopa taken by mouth must pass through the stomach and then via the pyloric valve into the small intestine before it can be absorbed into the blood stream. Unfortunately, the frequency of opening and closing the pyloric valve can vary anywhere from 30 to 90 minutes, depending on the amount of solid and liquid present in the stomach, the time of day, and the emotional state of the individual. In a continued effort to stabilize levodopa concentrations in the bloodstream, a number of strategies have been developed to try to overcome this variability in stomach "emptying" and subsequent levodopa absorption. One strategy takes advantage of the fact that levodopa is rapidly and completely absorbed in the duodenum, the first portion of the small intestine beyond the stomach. Bypassing the stomach and pyloric valve by delivering levodopa directly to the duodenum should eliminate the variability of stomach emptying and lead to a much more stable blood level of medication, which in turn should help reduce the "on-off" cycles. Most patients dislike this method of levodopa delivery because having a tube permanently inserted into the duodenum is uncomfortable and the pump that contains the levodopa solution is large and cumbersome.

Small trials of duodenal infusion showed this method of levodopa administration to be clearly superior to intermittent tablet therapy. Patients had longer functional "on" periods with fewer dyskinesias and "off" periods. This was the direct result of smoother blood levodopa levels and the ability to adjust the rate of levodopa infusion to each individual's clinical needs.

Some patients who completed this study continued to use the duodenal infusion method for control of their Parkinson's disease symptoms during the following 12–20 months. Mechanical difficulty with the pump or infusion tubing occasionally prevented use of the infusion system until repairs could be made. While experiencing this type of mechanical failure, one person noted that drinking the solution of medication at the same hourly rate pumped by the machine gave almost the same smooth result as from the pump itself. Other researchers had also previously observed that sipping a solution of levodopa gave better results than tablets taken by mouth.

Based on these reports, small pilot studies were conducted to test whether this method of administration of Sinemet® could be beneficial in patients with motor fluctuations. One pilot study that compared oral tablet therapy to intermittent liquid intake showed a significantly improved function with better "on," fewer dyskinesias, and fewer "off" periods with the liquid solution. Compared to tablet therapy, a solution of carbidopa/levodopa significantly reduced blood levodopa variability. The conclusion of this open study was that liquid CD/LD permitted patients to have better "on" time with fewer "off" periods by reducing the plasma levodopa variability and allowing better titration of levodopa to fit each patient's clinical needs.

Many people found the need to prepare the liquid solution cumbersome and tedious. Having to prepare the solution every day, having to remember to take it every hour, having to measure precisely the amount they drink, together with having to carry a flask around with them throughout the day, is simply too much for most people. For some, however, a solution of carbidopa/levodopa can provide unquestionable improvement and is a good alternative to duodenal infusions.

## ►ANTICHOLINERGIC DRUGS

Acetylcholine is a neurotransmitter that is involved in many brain functions, notably memory. In the striatum, the balance between the amounts of acetylcholine and dopamine is critical for smooth motor function. In Parkinson's disease, acetylcholine is unchanged but dopamine is decreased, thus tilting the balance. Drugs that block acetylcholine transmission restore this balance.

Anticholinergic agents such as trihexyphenidyl (Artane®), and benztropine (Cogentin®) were used extensively before the advent of levodopa therapy, but they are no longer considered drugs of first choice in the treatment of parkinsonian symptoms. Although clearly helpful, significant side effects limit their use, including memory impairment, urinary retention, and blurry vision. Elderly patients are especially likely to suffer from confusion and hallucinations. If anticholinergic drugs are abruptly discontinued, some patients develop severe worsening of their parkinsonian symptoms that is not easily treated with increased dopaminergic therapy. Therefore, anticholinergic drugs should be reserved for younger individuals who need additional therapy for tremor or dystonia. Interestingly, some younger patients seem to experience significantly enhanced benefit when anticholinergic drugs are used with high dose dopaminergic agonists.

## ►AMANTADINE (SYMMETREL®)

The mechanism of action of this drug remains elusive. Recent data suggest that it may antagonize a subclass of glutamate receptors. Amantadine can be very useful as initial therapy in some people. Unfortunately, identifying this responsive subgroup is a matter of trial and error. Side effects are usually mild, but can include leg and ankle edema (swelling), with or without livido reticularis (purplish or bluish mottling of the skin usually observed around the ankle, sometimes on the forearm), confusion, and hallucinations. Some people seem to lose benefit from the drug after a few months, but responsiveness can usually be regained following brief abstinence. Amantadine can significantly improve levodopa-induced dyskinesias in some patients when used as adjunct therapy (M. Kurth; personal observation). This drug is eliminated from the body only by the kidneys, and elderly patients with impaired renal function are at increased risk for side effects due to abnormal build-up of the drug; confusion and hallucinations may occur at high doses (300 mg a day).

## ▶ DOPAMINE RECEPTOR AGONISTS

As described in Chapter 1, substantia nigra nerve cells make dopamine, store it in small vesicles located in the nerve terminals, and release it into the synaptic cleft. On the other side of the cleft, neurons carry "receptors" to which dopamine binds (Figure 2.2). There are at least four different dopamine receptors, called D1, D2, D3, and D4 receptors. These receptors specifically recognize dopamine, and allow only dopamine to bind to them. Only the first three types have been found in the striatum. When dopamine binds to its receptors, a cascade of events is turned on that leads to dopamine's effects. Some drugs are dopamine "look-alikes" that bind to dopamine receptors and imitate its effects, turning on the cascade of events normally turned on by dopamine. Look-alikes that imitate dopamine are called dopamine receptor agonists.

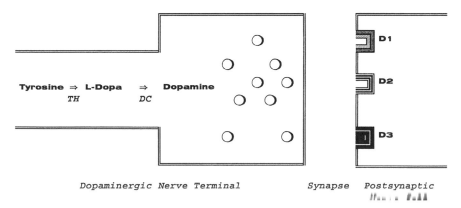

*Figure 2.2.* Schematic representation of a dopamine synapse. Dopamine is made in dopaminergic nerve terminals and stored in small vesicles. When it is released, it crosses the synapse and interacts with its receptors.

Some dopamine agonists bind to all dopamine receptors (like dopamine, they fit all the locks), whereas others bind mainly to one dopamine receptor.

The symptoms of Parkinson's disease are due to decreased levels of dopamine in the striatum and resultant decreased stimulation of dopamine receptors. Drugs that directly stimulate dopamine receptors imitate the effects of dopamine, and should therefore compensate for its loss. In fact, such drugs should even be better than levodopa in late-stage disease because they do not need to be converted into an active substance by dopaminergic nerve cells (levodopa must be converted into dopamine). The effect of dopamine agonists should therefore be independent of the number of nerve cells left in the substantia nigra and should remain the same in early- and late-stage disease.

Apomorphine is the oldest known dopamine agonist. It cannot be given by mouth, but it works almost as well as levodopa when infused intravenously. Unfortunately, other available dopamine agonists do not seem to work as well as levodopa. The reason for this disappointing result is unknown. Dopamine agonists are usually either prescribed alone in early-stage patients or are given in combination with levodopa when response to levodopa declines.

Two dopaminergic agonists are currently available in the United States. Bromcriptine (Parlodel®) was the first agent found to offer symptomatic relief both as adjunct therapy to levodopa and when given alone. Its major mechanism of action is a direct D2 dopamine receptor activation. When used alone, doses up to 120 mg may be needed to give an adequate response. Side effects include nausea, orthostatic hypotension (a drop of blood pressure when going from sitting to standing that can cause dizziness), and rarely livido reticularis. Increased dopaminergic stimulation can induce dyskinesias in patients on levodopa as well as hallucinations.

Pergolide (Permax®) is ten times more potent than bromocriptine at the D2 receptor and also stimulates D1 receptors. Its side effects are similar to those induced by bromocriptine, including rare instances of retroperitoneal fibrosis and livido reticularis. Pergolide has a longer half-life compared to bromocriptine (up to 24 hours versus a maximum of 8 to 12 hours). One animal study has demonstrated that pergolide reduces the loss of dopaminergic neurons due to aging, presumably by reducing oxidative stress and free radical overload incurred from dopamine metabolism. One study demonstrated a significant preference by patients for pergolide over bromocriptine. When used as the single agent in newly diagnosed patients with Parkinson's disease, 0.5 mg of pergolide is equivalent to 5 mg of bromocriptine and 100 mg of Sinemet®.

Two other dopamine agonists are available in Europe for the treatment of Parkinson's disease. Lisuride (Dopergine®) is a short-acting D2 agonist that is water soluble and can be infused continuously under the skin by a pump, and cabergoline is a very long-acting D2 agonist. Two other dopamine agonists, ropinerole and pramipexole, should soon become available in Europe and the United States. These drugs are described in more detail in Chapter 9.

Some authors suggest that early therapy with a dopamine receptor agonist is helpful in preventing the onset of late-stage motor complications, notably motor fluctuations. However, only about half of all patients can remain on an agonist alone for more than one year; the rest usually need the addition of levodopa to treat their symptoms adequately.

## ►WHEN SHOULD PATIENTS BEGIN SYMPTOMATIC THERAPY?

Age, occupation, and life-style needs are important points to keep in mind when deciding to initiate symptomatic therapy. Some people can tolerate a moderate tremor in their nondominant hand (i.e., the left hand in right-handers) without difficulty and may not need symptomatic treatment immediately. Others may elect to begin therapy for even mild symptoms of rigidity and slowness in order to perform their duties optimally in their work.

## ►SHOULD LEVODOPA THERAPY BE DELAYED TO PREVENT POTENTIAL TOXICITY?

Some neurologists believe that early therapy with levodopa may hasten the onset of complications such as motor fluctuations and dyskinesias. Some also argue that metabolism of levodopa and dopamine causes an increase in free radical load in the substantia nigra, thus accelerating disease progression. Others argue that there is no benefit to withholding levodopa therapy and that appropriate treatment with levodopa prolongs patient survival and improves quality of life. Some insist that patients who are treated early with levodopa therapy may actually develop fewer complications, including dyskinesias and motor fluctuations. Significant limitations in studies published to date make these conclusions somewhat tentative. Nevertheless, measurements of both quality and duration of life in available studies are convincing. Therefore, there is a consensus that people with Parkinson's disease suffering from any significant disability should not delay initiating levodopa therapy.

## ►NEUROPROTECTIVE THERAPY

The cause of Parkinson's disease remains unknown. One leading hypothesis states that Parkinson's disease is due to either external or internal stressors that increase the oxidative stress (due to toxic free radicals) on dopaminergic neurons. While not proven, this hypothesis is based on numerous studies that demonstrate evidence for oxidative damage in the remaining dopaminergic neurons. A serendipitous natural experiment in 1982 resulted in the discovery of the potent and selective neurotoxin 1-methyl-4-phenyl-1,2,3,6-tetrahydropyridine (MPTP). MPTP is a chemical byproduct generated during attempts to synthesize designer narcotics for sale to drug addicts. Use of this material by over 120 addicts resulted in several developing a severe parkinsonian syndrome that closely mimics idiopathic Parkinson's disease, including typical responses to dopaminergic replacement therapy. To be neurotoxic, MPTP must be activated by an enzyme called monoamine oxidase B (MAO-B) that normally degrades dopamine, and in doing so generates toxic free radicals and hydrogen peroxide as byproducts. Thus MAO-B may participate in the production of toxic products from both endogenous and exogenous sources. If this indeed is the case, then selective inhibition of this enzyme should reduce the rate of disease progression in patients with Parkinson's disease.

Based on this hypothesis, a large multicenter study was implemented in 1986—Deprenyl and Tocopherol Antioxidant Therapy of Parkinsonism (DATATOP). DATATOP studied 800 newly diagnosed parkinsonian patients for a two-year period to determine the effects of selegiline (an inhibitor of MAO-B) and tocopherol (vitamin E, which "scavenges" free radicals) on the need for patients to initiate levodopa replacement therapy. Patients on placebo reached this end point almost twice as fast as those receiving selegiline (selegiline, deprenyl, Eldepryl®). Tocopherol had no beneficial effect. While all patients reached the same objective end point, the conclusion that selegiline slowed the progression of the disease was subsequently extensively debated as due to properties of the drug that complicated interpretation of the study.

Although some subsequent studies found a small symptomatic effect with selegiline, all studies carried out in a rigorous fashion demonstrate reduced need for initiating levodopa therapy or show a reduction in progression of disease symptoms. One study went a step further and addressed the question of whether selegiline continues to reduce disease progression after symptomatic therapy (levodopa) is initiated. Patients on both levodopa and selegiline had significantly lower disability scores than those on levodopa and placebo, further supporting the hypothesis that selegiline slows the progression of Parkinson's disease.

Overall, selegiline appears to be well tolerated and to have few side effects in newly diagnosed patients. A previous history of peptic ulcer disease in patients is considered a relative contraindication because the drug increases the risk for this gastrointestinal complication. Nausea, lack of or decreased appetite, insomnia, and orthostatic hypotension are other relatively minor side effects. However, selegiline can significantly potentiate some side effects of levodopa therapy, including dyskinesia, gastrointestinal side effects, orthostatic hypotension, and—more likely in the older patient—confusion and hallucinations. Reducing levodopa dosage and increasing intervals between doses can reduce or eliminate these problems to a large degree.

A recent study conducted in the United Kingdom has called into question the safety of selegiline and suggested that it may shorten life expectancy in people with Parkinson's disease. The study followed two groups with early, mild Parkinson's disease for a little more than five years. Patients were treated either with levodopa alone or with levodopa and selegiline. There were 44 deaths in the group taking levodopa alone, as opposed to 76 deaths in the group taking levodopa and selegiline. This result was not influenced by age or gender. Disability scores were slightly higher in patients on levodopa alone, but severe motor complications were more frequent in the combined treatment group. The results came as a total surprise and were very different from previous results obtained with selegiline. Investigators stress that the precise cause of mortality in the group of patients receiving selegiline and levodopa needs to be carefully determined. A detailed review of the hospital charts of the patients who died during the study has begun. The increased mortality seen with selegiline could be due to the drug's effects on blood pressure and circulatory system, or it could be due to adverse interactions between selegiline and other drugs taken by the patients. Nothing is yet known about these possible interactions with other drugs. The average dose of levodopa was higher in the patients who did not take selegiline, but it seems unlikely that levodopa would reduce mortality. The scientific community stresses that confirmation of the results are needed, and this may come from current ongoing studies. Moreover, if the results were to be confirmed, it would be extremely helpful to find the biological explanation for this apparent increase in mortality.

## ►CONCLUSION

No treatment has yet been discovered that stops the progressive loss of nerve cells that characterizes Parkinson's disease. With the exception of selegiline, which may slow nerve cell loss (although this is controversial), all available treatments are directed at managing the symptoms of the disease. In this respect, levodopa remains the best treatment of the disease. However, the response to levodopa gradually becomes less satisfactory as the disease progresses. Early stage patients do very well on this medication; some even feel that their motor function has been restored to normal. The price to pay may be nausea, dizziness upon standing, or insomnia, However, disability breaks through over a period of years. This occurs not because levodopa loses efficacy, but rather because new symptoms that do not respond to levodopa make their appearance. Patients become sensitive to the short half-life of levodopa and start swinging on and off medication several times a day.

In theory, dopamine agonists should work as well as levodopa and should have the advantage of a longer half-life. In practice, however, dopamine agonists do not work as well as levodopa and are mainly useful when added on to it. Until a cure is found, patients need new drugs that better control late-stage symptoms and drugs that work as well as levodopa but have a longer half-life.

# 3

# Other Symptoms of Parkinson's Disease and Their Management

In addition to the classic parkinsonian triad of symptoms that are managed with levodopa, as discussed in Chapter 2, Parkinson's disease may involve a number of other symptoms. Some, such as gastrointestinal problems, appear to be in part due to the loss of dopamine neurons, while the cause of others is often unknown. Most can be successfully managed and produce little discomfort. This chapter discusses the most common symptoms seen in Parkinson's disease and their treatment.

## ▶DIFFICULTY WALKING

Impairment of gait gives parkinsonian patients their characteristic overall appearance. A narrow, shuffling gait and an associated stooped posture defines the fundamental "look" of Parkinson's disease. A further feature of this gait disorder is the phenomenon of "freezing," in which the feet and legs become completely immobilized or "frozen" to the ground. Tight spaces, doorways, elevators, rows of chairs or pews all increase the possibility of experiencing this problem. At first freezing may occur only when patients are experiencing an "off" period, (i.e., when their medication temporarily stops working). Later a significant number of individuals may experience freezing even while on optimal medical therapy.

# ▶ POSTURAL INSTABILITY

Balance problems are an important symptom of Parkinson's disease. In fact, loss of postural stability is a milestone in the progression of the illness. Some people suffer from postural instability early in the course of the disease, but the problem more often manifests itself later in the disease course.

The cause of postural instability differs in the early and late stages of the disease. Early in the course of the disease, some people may have postural instability because their bradykinesia and slowness in initiating movements make it difficult to maintain the center of gravity. In other words, they experience so much bradykinesia that they cannot initiate movements fast enough to catch themselves if they lose their center of balance. Because dopamine replacement therapy (i.e., levodopa contained in Sinemet® or Madopar®) significantly improves bradykinesia, patients often have essentially normal balance once levodopa treatment is initiated.

Unfortunately, most patients eventually develop difficulties with balance that cannot be corrected with medication. The underlying mechanism or even brain lesion that causes this difficulty is not yet known. Nevertheless, it can become a serious issue for many people. Some people may continue to have an excellent response to antiparkinsonian medication only to be plagued by balance problems that lead to numerous falls. When this occurs, they need to become aware of their limitations with regard to balance and must learn to use additional tools, such as canes or walkers, to avoid serious falls resulting in fractures of hips and other long bones.

# ▶ GASTROINTESTINAL PROBLEMS

The most common gastrointestinal problems in Parkinson's disease are difficulty swallowing, abnormal salivation and drooling, nausea, and constipation.

## Difficulty Swallowing

Swallowing requires the coordinated action of several groups of muscles and is a complex process that is normally performed without thinking about it. Since muscle strength and coordination are impaired in Parkinson's disease, it is not surprising if swallowing is compromised. The problem results from a lack of coordination between the muscles responsible for moving food particles to the back of the throat and into the esophagus. Swallowing difficulty can have serious and occasionally life-threatening consequences. It makes eating and taking medication difficult and is often the cause of choking. As a result, food can get into the lungs, where it causes inflammation, infection, and pneumonia.

### Abnormal Salivation and Drooling

Difficulty swallowing is also responsible for the impression that people with Parkinson's disease produce excess saliva and the resulting reaction of drooling. People with Parkinson's disease often think they make too much saliva. In reality, everyone produces saliva constantly and swallows it unconsciously. Drooling is simply one of the consequences of not swallowing at a normal rate. Levodopa therapy usually improves swallowing and reduces or eliminates drooling.

### Nausea

Drugs that stimulate dopamine transmission act not only in the striatum to normalize parkinsonian motor function, but also in the area postrema, the "vomiting center" of the brain to cause nausea and vomiting. Thus, it is not surprising that nausea is one of the most common side effects of antiparkinsonian drugs. The vomiting center typically adapts to dopamine-stimulating drugs, and nausea and vomiting gradually fade after a few months. However, this uncomfortable side effect persists in some people. Drugs to treat nausea and vomiting block a particular type of dopamine receptor, called D2, and cannot be used in those with Parkinson's disease because they cause the motor symptoms of the disease to worsen.

Domperidone (Motilium®) blocks these receptors. Because it is effective in the "vomiting center" but has hardly any effect in the striatum, it can prevent nausea without worsening the symptoms of Parkinson's disease. Domperidone is available in Europe and Canada, but not in the United States. Trials of the drug are ongoing in the United States for the treatment of gastrointestinal problems due to diabetes. The pharmaceutical company that makes domperidone hopes to obtain permission to make the drug commercially available within a few years. In the meantime, patients may be allowed to use the drug through a "compassionate use IND."

Very mild nausea may be responsible for the loss of appetite so often reported by people with Parkinson's disease, and domperidone may help restore a normal appetite. Since people with Parkinson's disease have trouble eating for many other reasons, it may be important to relieve at least one cause of the problem. In this respect, domperidone could be a useful adjunct to antiparkinsonian treatment.

Many investigators believe that nausea is not only a side effect of antiparkinsonian drugs, but a symptom of the disease due to delayed gastric emptying. Like swallowing, moving food from the stomach into the intestines requires a well-coordinated sequence of muscle movements, and this sequence appears to be disrupted and slowed in Parkinson's disease. Acceleration of stomach emptying can be promoted by certain medications that block the D2 receptor in the gut, but they also block D2 receptors in the brain and worsen the signs and symptoms of Parkinson's disease. Because domperidone enters the striatum only minimally, it improves stomach emptying without worsening the signs of Parkinson's disease. Thus domperidone can be beneficial at two levels.

Another drug, Cisapride (Propulsid®), is commercially available in the United States and is helpful in accelerating gastric emptying in patients with Parkinson's disease. It may partially alleviate nausea and loss of appetite, but it does not have any beneficial effect on the brain vomiting center.

### Constipation

Slowness of movement seems to affect the bowel as it does the rest of the body, and chronic constipation is a common problem in Parkinson's disease. Most often it is only a nuisance and responds to common remedies such as eating more fiber, increasing fluid intake, and physical exercise. It is sometimes more serious and requires medical treatment. Very rarely, severe constipation is associated with an enlargement of the colon that can result in an obstruction that requires surgery.

Constipation in its milder forms is often overlooked, perhaps because it is so poorly understood. Until a few years ago it was commonly accepted that constipation was a side effect of antiparkinsonian medications and simply had to be tolerated. This view has now been called into question. While it is certainly true that anticholinergic drugs and some antidepressant drugs cause constipation, this does not seem to be the case for other antiparkinsonian drugs. Many investigators now believe that constipation is actually a symptom of the disease, and that it may be related to the selective loss of dopamine-producing nerve cells that surround the bowel and control bowel muscles.

Laxatives will be needed if dietary measures are not sufficient to prevent constipation. This should begin with "bulk" laxatives such as Metamucil® that retain water in the stool. A tablespoonful per day stirred in a glass of water may be sufficient. Another useful substance is the stool softener dioctyl sodium sulfosuccinate (docusate sodium) found in many over-the-counter preparations. If none of these measures work, "irritant" laxatives may be used. Patients should first try mild irritants such as bisacodyl (Dulcolax®).

Acetylcholine is a neurotransmitter that causes the heart to beat faster, the stomach to secrete acid juices, the bowel to move faster, and saliva to be produced. It also plays a central role in memory. By its action on the bowel, acetylcholine opposes constipation. Drugs that stimulate acetylcholine receptors or increase acetylcholine transmission should therefore be helpful in the treatment of constipation. However, these drugs have widespread effects that makes their use impractical. Cisapride (Propulsid®) seems to increase acetylcholine concentrations only in the bowel. Thus, in addition to its effects on gastric emptying, cisapride accelerates intestinal transit time in patients with Parkinson's disease and improves symptoms of constipation without causing either diarrhea or a worsening of the motor symptoms of Parkinson's disease.

### Slow Intestinal Transit Causes Unpredictable Levodopa Absorption

Levodopa (Sinemet® or Madopar®) taken by mouth has several barriers to cross before it can enter the brain, the first being the stomach itself. Erratic emptying of the stomach may contribute to poor clinical response and motor fluctuations. Patients with slow gastric emptying keep medication in their stomach for many hours and then deliver significant amounts of levodopa erratically to the bowel several hours after its oral intake. This produces an unpredictable response, or even a lack of response, when the stomach is closed. Conversely, dyskinesias can occur several hours after medication intake, when the stomach suddenly opens and dumps excessive medication into the small intestine. The observation that administration of levodopa by a duodenal tube (directly into the small intestine) minimizes response fluctuations proves that irregular absorption is in part responsible for unpredictable responses to levodopa.

By normalizing gastric emptying, cisapride increases the absorption of levodopa from the bowel, as judged by plasma concentrations of levodopa in the bloodstream. In keeping with this improved absorption, cisapride enhances response to treatment in patients with delayed gastric emptying. In these patients, cisapride also decreases the latency of onset of therapeutic benefit from levodopa and improves the predictability of the response to treatment. It therefore appears to be a useful add-on medication for patients with Parkinson's disease and slow gastric emptying.

## ▶ URINARY URGENCY

Bladder problems are common in patients with Parkinson's disease. The most usual is an urge to void even when the bladder is not full. This symptom can be particularly annoying at night, causing frequent awakening and the need to get up. It is usually relieved by anticholinergic drugs. Urologists often prescribe oxybutynin chloride (Ditropan®). Less often, patients with Parkinson's disease have trouble voiding, urination is slowed, and the bladder is incompletely emptied, causing the need to void frequently. This symptom is also particularly disturbing at night. Serious disturbance of bladder function are rare in Parkinson's disease. If they occur, another cause should be suspected, and patients should consult their physician. Further tests may be needed. Prostate enlargement or infection of the bladder are often the cause of urinary problems.

## ►SLEEP DISORDERS

People with Parkinson's disease seem to have more problems with sleeping than the general population. This is not simply explained by the fact that Parkinson's disease occurs late in life and that sleep disorders are more common with aging. Sleep problems may be partly due to the loss of serotonin nerve cells in the brainstem. People with Parkinson's disease may experience difficulty falling asleep or staying asleep, frequent unexplained awakenings, a sense of disturbed or non-restful sleep, and excessive sleepiness during the day. Although these symptoms may in part be the consequence of aging, they can also be due to Parkinson's disease or antiparkinsonian medications.

### Sleep Problems Related to Antiparkinsonian Medication

Drugs that increase dopamine transmission—as most antiparkinsonian drugs do—can cause difficulty falling asleep, vivid dreaming, or abnormal involuntary movements during the night. Nightmares rather than simple vivid dreaming may also occur, and patients may occasionally "act out" their nightmares—shouting, kicking, grabbing, punching, or jumping out of bed. Sleep terrors are also seen in people who have Parkinson's disease: typically, they wake with a sense of terror but do not recall a vivid dream. Reducing the evening dose of antiparkinsonian medication is usually helpful when such side effects occur. They are more pronounced at the beginning of treatment and tend to wane after a few weeks.

Sleep problems are sometimes due to insufficient medication, so that symptoms return during the night. Patients wake up because they have trouble rolling over in bed. More distressingly, they may have difficulty getting out of bed to go to the toilet, which then causes them to become fully awake. The evening dose of antiparkinsonian medication must be carefully adjusted. Too high a dose causes insomnia; too small a dose leads to uncomfortable and worrisome situations during the night.

### Sleep Problems Caused by Parkinson's Disease

Even when antiparkinsonian medication is well adjusted, sleep is often disturbed due to a direct effect of Parkinson's disease on sleep. Patients frequently complain of unexplained awakenings, a loss of the normal restorative properties of sleep, or even disturbances in normal sleep rhythms.

People with Parkinson's disease often have trouble falling asleep. This can be due to medical conditions such as anxiety, depression, or breathing problems, but may also be due to motor problems. Some patients experience an unpleasant sensation in their legs as they try to fall asleep, with an urge to move for relief. This "restless leg syndrome" may be associated with involuntary leg jerks called myoclonus, which occur during sleep and can awaken them. In others, sleep is disturbed by painful leg cramps.

Some people have no trouble falling asleep but complain of frequent, unexplained awakenings during the night or of waking earlier than they would like. Alcohol (even in moderate amounts at night), caffeine, and nicotine can all cause this type of insomnia. Early morning awakening is also typical of depression.

Some people with Parkinson's disease suffer from disturbances in the sleep/wake cycle. They feel sleepy in the early evening and wake up too early in the morning. Because they get a full night's sleep if they go to bed early, their problem is not insomnia, but rather that the sleep cycle has shifted in a fashion similar to jet lag. Some investigators suggest that melatonin, which can normalize sleep cycles in travelers, might have the same effect in "shifted" patients. Other disturbances in the sleep/wake cycle consist of frequent daytime naps and an inability to sleep normally at night.

### Sleep Management

People who have sleep difficulties should follow a few simple guidelines that may be sufficient to promote a better sleep pattern. The following are a few of the many rules of good sleep hygiene.

- Develop regular bedtime habits. Get up at the same time each day even if you have not slept and feel tired.
- If naps are helpful, they should be taken daily. Occasional napping usually causes people to sleep less well at night.
- If you wake up during the night, try to remain in bed and relax. If you feel yourself becoming tense, try to do something relaxing.
- Exercise during the day is very important to develop a good night's sleep. The many benefits of exercise are detailed in Chapter 5. Exercise should be avoided in the evening because of its stimulating effects.
- Save your bedroom for sleep, and try not to sleep anywhere else. This will condition your body to associate the bedroom with sleep.
- Reduce fluids after dinner to avoid the need to get up during the night.
- Avoid coffee, tea, chocolate, and cola in the late afternoon. Some people find they need to avoid these drinks from noon onwards.
- Avoid late evening alcohol consumption. Alcohol has a double effect on sleep. It produces sleepiness when it first enters the brain, but has a short half-life and causes people to wake up when its effects wear off.

People vary tremendously as far as sleep is concerned. What promotes sleep for one person may cause insomnia in another. Individuals should therefore find what suits them best and do it.

### The Medical Evaluation and Treatment of Sleep Disorders

Medical evaluation may be needed if symptoms of sleep disturbance persist despite a well-followed and sound sleep program. Sleep specialists usually start by prescribing a medication to treat insomnia. Since one of the frequent causes of sleep problems is depression, they often begin by giving patients a sedating antidepressant such as trazodone. If anxiety seems to be the principal reason for insomnia, treatment with an anti-anxiety drug such as clonazepam may be warranted.

The initial medical evaluation may suggest a problem that requires further testing in a sleep disorder center, which usually involves spending the night in the sleep laboratory. The patient's sleep is monitored so events such as sleep apnea or abnormal movements can be identified. Sleep testing usually leads to a correct diagnosis and specific treatment recommendations.

People who have difficulty sleeping should be aware that there are many available treatments and the chances are high that normal sleep can be restored.

## ►BREATHING DIFFICULTIES

Respiratory problems are common in Parkinson's disease. They are mainly due to lack of coordination between the two groups of muscles involved in breathing. One group moves the chest, allowing it to propel air in and out of the lungs, including the diaphragm and the muscles lying between the ribs, which help form the chest wall. A second group of muscles controls the larynx, the inlet to the lungs.

Rigidity of the chest wall muscles makes deep breathing difficult. Levodopa decreases this rigidity and improves respiration. The muscles of the chest wall, like those elsewhere in the body, are weakened by inactivity and strengthened by work. Work for the respiratory muscles occurs in the process of deep breathing, such as is required by high levels of physical activity. Unfortunately, people with Parkinson's disease tend to give up physical exercise. Clearly, however, exercise is essential for their lungs (and for many other reasons).

Another cause of breathing problems is the improper opening of the larynx. Just inside the larynx are the vocal cords, and normal breathing requires that they be kept open. This is accomplished by a single pair of small muscles. Tremors, spasms, impaired coordination, and abnormal involuntary movements (dyskinesias) prevent these muscles from properly opening the larynx. Thus, people with Parkinson's disease struggle with insufficient coordination of their breathing muscles (diaphragm and chest wall) and insufficient opening of the pipe that allows air to flow into the lungs.

In some, problems with opening of the larynx occur mainly at night, intermittently shutting off air flow and depriving the brain and heart of oxygen. This can be the cause of frequent awakenings. The most common problem is sleep apnea, characterized by frequent pauses in breathing during sleep. It is most often caused by the collapse of tissue within the throat. This form of sleep apnea is characterized by loud snoring, interrupted by pauses in breathing. Other forms of sleep apnea are not associated with collapse of tissue within the throat, and snoring is often absent. People with sleep apnea sometimes wake up with a choking or gasping sensation, but they usually are not aware of their problem and the disorder is reported by their bed partners. The quality of sleep is disturbed, and patients may experience increased sleepiness during the day.

Respiratory problems can be made worse by swallowing difficulties. Patients with incoordinated swallowing muscles may experience severe problems with choking. Incoordination of swallowing can cause small amounts of liquid and food to pass into the larynx and be aspirated into the lungs. Inflammation and even infection can develop, especially in those who do not take deep breaths.

There is usually plenty of warning that problems with the opening of the larynx are developing. People may find that they often run out of breath while talking or that they frequently gasp for air. Others may experience a coarsening hoarseness or high-pitched sound with breathing called stridor, the telltale sign of vocal cord closure. When it occurs at night, stridor can be mistaken for simple snoring, but the sounds of snoring and stridor are different. Snoring sounds emanate from the nose and the back of the throat and tend to be coarse, tremorous, and loud. Stridor sounds are high-pitched and more of a struggling wheeze. When stridor occurs, it becomes relatively urgent to seek medical attention.

A number of fairly simple tests are used to evaluate a breathing problem. They usually involve little discomfort or risk to the patient and lead to accurate diagnosis and appropriate treatment.

## ►SPEECH DIFFICULTIES

Changes in speech are a common symptom of Parkinson's disease. In many people speech is not affected for several years, but in others it is affected early in the course of the disease. The first change is usually a tendency to speak softly. Increased stiffness in the muscles surrounding the vocal cords is a contributing factor to speech difficulties. Another characteristic change in speech is the tendency to talk in a monotone fashion—the natural tonal variation and rhythm of speech is lost. Some patients speak rapidly, crowding their words together. Imprecise articulation is also frequent. The reasons for such changes are still incompletely understood. These changes in speech may be improved by antiparkinsonian medication

Traditional speech therapy is not very helpful. Recently a type of voice therapy known as the Lee Silverman Voice Treatment (LSVT) was developed specifically for Parkinson's disease. It consists of four 50–60 minute sessions a week for a total of 16 sessions in one month. It improves vocal intensity (loudness), intonation, vocal steadiness, and speech intelligibility. Patients who received LSVT say they speak more often and more confidently because people understand them better. Simple things can also be helpful, such as exercising the voice every day by reading aloud, singing, yelling, and shouting.

It is helpful to simply acknowledge that the problem exists and adapt to it. People should try to avoid making long sentences because the voice tends to become softer at their end. They should concentrate on talking slowly. All this is easier said than done, but exercise is useful. Another helpful strategy is to avoid talking in loud and noisy places or in a room where a television, radio, or dishwasher is on. Finally, people should not hesitate to inform those with whom they are speaking that they have a speech problem and make them feel free to interrupt when they do not understand. This can help communication a great deal by relieving the anxiety of the listener. If a soft voice is a major problem, devices that accurately amplify the human voice can be found at reasonable prices in electronics shops or from the local telephone company. Advances in technology have allowed for better and smaller devices.

Speech difficulties do not always fully respond to antiparkinsonian medication and may contribute to the isolation of the patient by making communication difficult. The loss of facial expressive movements and hand gestures during speech can further decrease the ability to communicate. Certain types of speech therapy can be quite useful. Recognizing the problem and avoiding situations that make it worse can also help.

## ►LOW BLOOD PRESSURE

Most people with Parkinson's disease have normal blood pressure. Some have normal blood pressure when they are sitting or lying down but pressure drops when they stand up, a problem called *postural hypotension*. If the blood pressure is sufficiently low, people experience weakness, dizziness, lightheadedness, and faintness, especially when first arising after standing or lying down. These symptoms occur because arterial pressure is not high enough to send enough blood (and therefore oxygen) to the brain. Levodopa and drugs that stimulate dopamine receptors also cause postural hypotension, and in some people the combined effects of the disease and treatment on blood pressure can be quite handicapping.

Several treatments are available, including salt tablets, fluorohydrocortisone, caffeine, ergots, nasal antidiuretic hormone, and, if necessary, midodrine, a drug that causes blood vessels to contract and thereby increases blood pressure. A number of mechanical aids can also be useful to counter orthostatic hypotension, including elastic stockings (support hose) that must be put on in the morning before getting up, raising the head of the bed at night by three to four inches, and drinking plenty of fluids.

## ▶ DEPRESSION

Depression affects the way we feel and think, with negative feelings and pessimistic thoughts central symptoms of the illness. It is one of the most common medical conditions, and up to 25 percent of all Americans suffer from depression at least once in their lives. Typical signs of depression include:

- An inability to experience pleasure;
- Loss of interest in activities that were previously enjoyed;
- An inability to feel enthusiasm about anything;
- Loss of hope and a conviction that things will never improve;
- Low self-esteem and poor self-image;
- A tendency to become angry for apparently minor reasons or to have feelings easily hurt;
- A loss of energy and feelings of tiredness;
- Difficulty concentrating and loss of memory; elderly people often become afraid of having Alzheimer's disease;
- Problems with sleep, including waking up very early in the morning without being able to get back to sleep, problems in falling asleep, and frequent awakenings during the night.

Up to half of all people diagnosed with Parkinson's disease experience depression severe enough to seek medical attention. Moreover, Parkinson's disease is often initially misdiagnosed as depression because many of the symptoms overlap. Depressed people may appear sad or expressionless, think slowly, act slowly, speak slower—even memory may be impaired. However, depression does not cause rigidity, tremor, or other neurologic findings that must be present to diagnose Parkinson's disease, and the development of obvious motor symptoms eventually leads to the correct diagnosis and therapy.

### The Neurochemistry of Depression

It is not surprising that depression and Parkinson's disease resemble each other in so many ways once the common basis of their neurochemistry is understood. Parkinson's disease results from the loss of dopamine-producing neurons in the substantia nigra that are involved in the regulation of voluntary movement. Dopamine-producing neurons in different brain areas are involved in processing pleasure and mood, feelings that are affected in depression. The fact that mood swings often parallel motor fluctuations in people with Parkinson's disease further reinforces the notion that dopamine is involved in mood. Patients may alternate between feelings of despair when "off" to an almost euphoric sense of well-being when levodopa takes effect.

Not surprisingly, drugs that increase dopamine transmission also improve mood. Cocaine is the best known and most specific of the dopamine re-uptake blockers. It strongly potentiates the effects of dopamine, leading to the sense of euphoria and well-being craved by those who use it. Its potentiation of dopamine transmission suggests that cocaine might help patients with Parkinson's disease, but in fact it has only marginal benefit, probably because cocaine lacks specificity for any area of the brain. Cocaine is not helpful for the treatment of depression either, probably because the neurochemistry of depression involves more than just dopamine.

The neurochemical cause of depression is complex, and the exact role of dopamine in depression and mood is not fully understood. Replacing dopamine or increasing its effect in the brain is not sufficient to reverse classic depression. Another important neurotransmitter, serotonin, is now the major focus of attempts to understand depression and sleep/wake abnormalities. Serotonin is made by neurons within the brainstem. These neurons often are affected by Parkinson's disease but at a slower rate and later in the course of the illness than the cells of the substantia nigra. This loss of serotonin-producing neurons may be directly responsible for the sleep problems experienced by many Parkinsonian patients; whether it also favors depression is unclear.

Research on the mechanism of action of antidepressant medications also implicates serotonin as central to the neurochemistry of depression because all antidepressants substantially block its re-uptake. The newest and most potent antidepressants are selective serotonin re-uptake inhibitors (SSRIs); Prozac® was the first of these. None of these effective, safe, and useful medications has any significant effect on the dopamine neurotransmitter system, yet in patients with Parkinson's disease they usually alleviate depression and increase energy within a few weeks. This suggests that depression in people with Parkinson's disease is no different from "regular" depression and involves decreased concentrations of serotonin in certain areas of the brain.

### Diagnosis of Depression

There are many effective treatments for depression, and it is important to recognize its early signs. What symptoms indicate that a person with Parkinson's disease is suffering from more than just the "blues" and might benefit from antidepressant medication? It is not sufficient to simply refer to the list of symptoms that identify depression in otherwise healthy individuals because many of the same symptoms can be due to Parkinson's disease. It is important to discuss feelings of hopelessness, lack of energy, changes in relationships, and other less obvious areas affected by depression in an open and honest manner with one's family and doctor. The persistence of any of the following symptoms for more than a few weeks indicates that antidepressant treatment may be needed.

- Feelings of worthlessness, helplessness, or hopelessness that never seem to abate;
- Lack of interest in things that formerly gave pleasure;
- Major changes in appetite leading to significant weight gain or loss;
- Change in sleep habits out of proportion to the usual difficulties caused by Parkinson's disease itself;
- A desire to be alone and avoid other people even though symptoms of Parkinson's disease have not significantly changed;
- Becoming easily irritated by little things, tearful for no apparent reason, or more difficult to be with;
- Feelings that one might be better off dead or an inability to foresee a future.

### Treatment of Depression

Antidepressant therapy must be individualized to minimize side effects and optimize the chance of rapid recovery. Antidepressants usually take up to three weeks to have an effect. Most specialists agree that antidepressant therapy should be continued for at least six months, even if the patient is doing well. Some people do not respond to the first antidepressant they are given, and after six to eight weeks another type of medication will be prescribed. People should not be discouraged when this happens; depression is among the most treatable of medical disorders.

Specialists who treat depression in people with Parkinson's disease often recommend SSRIs because the older tricyclic antidepressants have significant anticholinergic effects that can lead to confusion or even hallucinations, particularly in elderly patients. However, the sedating effects of the tricylic antidepressants may be useful in patients who suffer from a significant sleep disorder. A good compromise that often works well is to combine the tricyclic antidepressant trazodone with an SSRI. Trazodone alone is not a very potent antidepressant, but it is much more sedating that the SSRIs and can be useful as a nighttime sleep aid. It is less likely to cause confusion or hallucinations. Buproprion, an unusual antidepressant that is chemically unrelated to any other agent, inhibits dopamine uptake and improves both depression and motor performance.

### DOs and DON'Ts During Antidepressant Therapy

- Alcohol should be avoided because it increases drowsiness and worsens depression.
- Driving should be avoided at the start of treatment with a sedating antidepressant.
- All antihistamines (the ingredients of many cold tablets) must be avoided because they increase the sedating action of antidepressants.
- Exercise and a balanced diet help fight depression and their use should not be overlooked.
- Sleep is important for depressed patients but it is often compromised. Depressed patients should not hesitate to discuss their sleep problems with their physicians.

Psychotherapy is a useful adjunct in managing depression. The root of depression in people who have medical problems is often grief over the loss of good health and difficulty accepting the problems that come with illness. Psychotherapy alone is not recommended for the treatment of depression, and most specialists believe that psychotherapy should only be started once the antidepressants have begun to work. Psychotherapy helps both to consolidate the effects of antidepressant medications and to prevent relapses, but alone it cannot cure an episode of depression.

## ►FATIGUE

People with Parkinson's disease often complain of feeling tired, described in simple terms such as "I tire so easily, Doctor" or "I can barely walk a block without feeling exhausted." The perception of fatigue is troublesome and interferes with everyday activities.

Muscle strength does not seem to be altered in proportion to the complaint of tiring easily, and often there is no direct relationship between reports of tiredness and severity of disease. Some investigators have found abnormalities in the generation of energy in the muscles of patients with Parkinson's disease and have suggested that this could be the cause of fatigue. Others are of the opinion that easy tiring is due to slowness of movement and difficulty stopping one movement in order to start the next one. People with Parkinson's disease have to concentrate much more than normal to accomplish apparently simple tasks such as walking. The easy fatigability of people with Parkinson's disease may be linked to the exaggerated mental efforts required to perform motor tasks.

A recent study attempted to determine whether easy tiring was due to a problem of muscle or brain. The results suggested that most of the problem resided in the brain and could be related to bradykinesia (slowness of movement). Levodopa treatment usually helps reduce fatigue, presumably by decreasing bradykinesia and muscle stiffness.

## ►ABNORMAL TEMPERATURE PERCEPTION AND EXCESSIVE SWEATING

People with Parkinson's disease often have disturbed perception of temperature. The most common is a sense of heat, which may occur in up to 50 percent of those with the disorder. This may be minor, only causing a dislike of warm rooms, or it may be a source of considerable discomfort. Others may have an abnormal sensation of cold and always feels chilly, or the sensations of cold and heat may alternate. Sensations of warmth are frequently accompanied by increased perspiration, which may be profuse.

These symptoms are still only poorly understood. Sweating plays an essential role in maintaining body temperature. Excessive sweating is a common manifestation of Parkinson's disease, which may explain the abnormal perception of temperature. It can be localized to one part of the body, but it is usually generalized. It typically occurs in irregular bursts, often when the effects of levodopa wear off.

Most people with Parkinson's disease experience sweating disturbances, but rather than increased sweating the disease process may actually involve decreased sweating that worsens with advancing disease. The bursts of increased sweating may be an attempt to compensate for chronic, insufficient sweating. The mechanism involved in this loss of normal sweating is unknown, and there is as yet no specific treatment for this annoying symptom. Antiparkinsonian medication partially normalizes sweating.

Increases in oiliness and sweating can lead to increased deposits of bacteria and risk of skin infections and rashes. The most common skin changes are increased oil secretion and a form of acne that, when they occur together, is called *seborrheic dermatitis*. Patients often complain of these changes affecting their scalp and hair. When extremely bothersome, they can be treated with special soaps, shampoos, and lotions obtained from a dermatologist.

## ▶ SEXUALITY

People with Parkinson's disease rarely discuss sexual difficulties with their physicians, for reasons that may primarily be due to mutual reticence and cultural factors. Little is presently known about sexual dysfunction in women with Parkinson's disease, but it is known that a wide variety of drugs used to treat the various symptoms of Parkinson's disease may interfere with erectile function in men. Depression may also affect sexual function, primarily the experience of desire.

If an adjustment in medications does not improve sexual function, it may be worthwhile to have a urologic and endocrine evaluation. A number of pharmacologic treatments may be useful. Previously untreated patients may find that levodopa therapy improves sexual function, most likely due to an improvement in motor function as well as an increase in sexual desire.

# 4
# *Surgical Treatment*

Neurosurgeons have long tried to treat Parkinson's disease by destroying certain specific groups of nerve cells. Early results were often disappointing and serious complications were frequent. These poor results occurred because the technology to accurately place lesions did not yet exist and the instruments used destroyed too much tissue. After levodopa therapy was introduced, its benefits were so remarkable that neurosurgery was reserved only for patients who tolerated levodopa poorly or who had persistent tremor despite optimal drug treatment. Only a small number of neurosurgeons continued to develop surgical procedures, and they gradually improved their techniques.

Current surgical results are far superior to those using earlier techniques. The risk of destroying the wrong brain region has been substantially decreased. Also contributing to a renewed interest in surgical approaches to the management of Parkinson's disease is the emergence of long-term motor complications with levodopa treatment, such as end-of-dose wearing-off and dyskinesias, which do not respond well to levodopa. End-of-dose wearing-off is also unresponsive to surgery, but dyskinesias are among the symptoms that respond best.

The first major improvement in surgical techniques was the introduction of stereotactic procedures, in which long needle-like probes are lowered into the brain area to be ablated. Once the probe is in place, a radio frequency is applied to the tip of the needle to heat the surrounding area and destroy the overactive neurons. This method is similar to the way microwaves heat water.

The next major improvement came from the field of radiology, with the development of techniques that link radiologic procedures to sophisticated computers, such as CT scan (computerized x-ray tomography or CAT scan) and MRI (magnetic resonance imaging). These help to localize brain areas with great precision and allow the surgeon to calculate accurately and quickly the angles at which the surgical probe should be lowered. Probes can now be positioned with great accuracy.

Further improvement in lesion placement was made by recording the electrical activity of the nerve cells at the tip of the probe. Nerve cells are continually active and areas of the brain have specific "firing" patterns; for example, the firing pattern of striatal cells is unlike that of cells in the globus pallidum. The electrical activity at the tip of the probe is transformed into noise, which sounds a bit like static on a radio. To locate pallidal nerve cells, the neurosurgeon slowly lowers the probe into the deep regions of the brain as directed by the computer, "listening" until the characteristic firing of the globus pallidum cells is heard. The surgeon can then move the probe cautiously to find the boundaries of the globus pallidum, so as to place the lesion in the middle of the area to be removed, not near the boundaries where damage could overlap into other areas.

## ►WHAT NEURONS SHOULD BE DESTROYED?

Surgery for Parkinson's disease targets those brain areas that receive input from the striatum (Figure 4.1). In parkinsonian monkeys, immediate relief of all parkinsonian symptoms follows destruction of the subthalamic nucleus (STN), which "drives" the internal part of the globus pallidum (GPi). However, the STN is a small structure and is not an ideal target for surgery. Earlier studies showed that destruction of the GPi, a procedure referred to as *pallidotomy*, could be extremely helpful for patients, but, as noted previously, it had been plagued by a high incidence of complications.

## ►RISKS AND BENEFITS OF PALLIDOTOMY

Although new technology has simplified pallidotomy and lessened the risks associated with the procedure, complications occur in about one of ten operations. One major risk is that the surgical probe may strike a blood vessel and cause bleeding and clotting, resulting in a slight stroke. Other risks

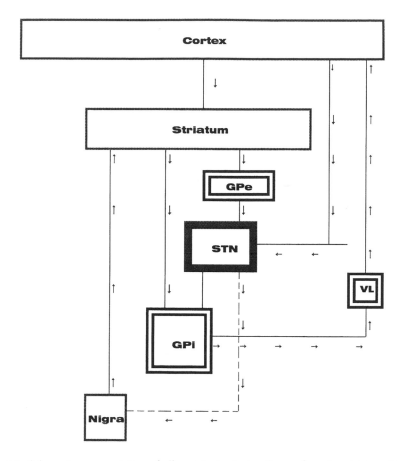

*Figure 4.1.* Schematic representation of efferent (outgoing) pathways from the striatum. Neurons in the substantia nigra (nigra) that deliver dopamine to the striatum die as a result of Parkinson's disease. Decreased levels of dopamine in the striatum are the cause of increased activity in the GPi (internal segment globus pallidum) and in the STN (subthalamic nucleus). VL: ventrolateral nucleus of thalamus; GPe: external segment pallidum.

linked to damage of adjacent brain structures are visual loss and decreased strength of the muscles of the face, arm, and leg.

Such risks may be worth taking if surgery offers dramatic improvement from the disabling symptoms of Parkinson's disease. Is there evidence of long-lasting symptomatic relief after this procedure? Several centers in the United States have developed the necessary tools and skills to perform pallidotomy for Parkinson's disease in a well-controlled manner. The present view is that pallidotomy is beneficial for some but not all patients.

The most spectacular effect of pallidotomy is the almost complete elimination of peak-dose dyskinesias. Slowness of movement (bradykinesia) and tremor are somewhat improved, mainly on the side opposite to the pallidotomy. Painful dystonia (cramps) induced by levodopa also seems to benefit from the procedure, but problems with balance and gait are essentially unrelieved. Age appears to be important, with younger patients seeming to benefit most. Pallidotomy therefore tends to be reserved for people under the age of 70 who are not responding well to levodopa and who have motor fluctuations, especially peak-dose dyskinesias. Pallidotomy also improves the response to antiparkinsonian medication. Only a few patients need less medication following surgery, and many actually take more because they no longer experience disabling peak-dose dyskinesias. While patients have an improved quality of life after pallidotomy, patients and physicians agree that the disease is still present and progressing.

The follow-up of more than 60 pallidotomies done at Emory University confirmed that its benefit is age-related. When measuring symptoms of Parkinson's disease in patients off all medications and looking at pre- and post-operative scores, younger patients clearly had a significantly greater improvement in symptoms than older ones. Patients over age 70 showed only mild improvement. In conclusion, younger patients may expect relief of parkinsonian symptoms and decreased severity of medication-induced side effects after pallidotomy. However, the disease will continue to have persistent slow progression. Older patients seem to have a shorter response to surgical therapy and more rapid disease progression. Why the outcome of the procedure is so age-dependent is unclear. Perhaps other changes in the brain that are age-related become more important, or perhaps Parkinson's disease differs in older and younger patients.

Little is known about the effects of pallidotomy on the long-term course of Parkinson's disease. One report shows progression of disease on the side unaffected by pallidotomy, progression of generalized slowness, and continued loss of regulation of the autonomic nervous system, which regulates functions such as blood pressure and sweating. Thus, patients continue to lose functionality as the disease slowly progresses.

## ►BILATERAL PALLIDOTOMY

Most pallidotomies are unilateral, or done only on one side of the brain. The results of the few bilateral procedures that have been performed have usually been disappointing. There has been a high rate of serious complications, such that this procedure should only be considered in extreme cases. These disappointing results may be explained by the function of the GPi, a brain region that acts rather like a "brake" on motor activity. When concentrations of dopamine decrease in the striatum, the activity of the GPi increases and consequently so does the brake on motor activity. Many believe that the activity of the GPi increases slowly and steadily with disease progression, so that patients have to fight a tighter and tighter brake. For a person with Parkinson's disease, trying to move becomes like trying to drive a car with the brakes on—movement is slow, difficult, and jerky. Destruction of the GPi on one side of the brain (unilateral pallidotomy) partially releases the brake on motor activity. Bilateral pallidotomy completely releases it, and the result may be analogous to trying to drive a car with no brakes at all.

## ►FURTHER EVALUATION OF PALLIDOTOMY IS NEEDED

Although pallidotomy can transform the lives of some patients, it is not a universal treatment for Parkinson's disease. Those who benefit most from the procedure are people with severe peak-dose dyskinesias. Perhaps pallidotomy might also benefit patients with other symptoms that do not respond well to levodopa. More research is needed to determine what pallidotomy might offer patients who suffer from problems such as medication-induced hallucinations, mild dementia, and severe speech or swallowing problems. The next few years will be instructive as investigators begin to compare their results and openly discuss the risks and benefits of such an invasive, yet potentially beneficial, technique. Such data will also allow a comparison of pallidotomy with the increasing number of excellent and safe medical therapies that are expected to become available.

## ►HIGH FREQUENCY ELECTRICAL STIMULATION

The principle underlying this procedure is based on the observation that nerve cells subjected to high frequency electrical stimulation "freeze" and become essentially paralyzed. High frequency electrical stimulation of nerves cells might thus be a viable alternative to surgery. The final result is the same, but the procedure is reversible when the stimulation is turned off. High frequency electrical stimulation of the globus pallidum therefore has the same effects as pallidotomy, with the advantage of not destroying nerve cells.

To perform high frequency electrical stimulation, fine wire electrodes are implanted into the globus pallidum using the same radiologic techniques as for pallidotomy. As the electrodes are lowered into the deep regions of the brain, the surgeon listens to the firing patterns of nerve cells to accurately place the high frequency electrical stimulation. Once placed, the electrode is left in the globus pallidum and connected to a battery-driven stimulator that patients can turn on or off when they wish. When the stimulator is on, high frequency electrical currents pass through the globus pallidum to "paralyze" the nerve cells, and beneficial effects occur within less than a minute.

Various brain areas can be stimulated; for example, electrical stimulation of the STN is effective on bradykinesia and rigidity. High frequency electrical stimulation of the GPi carries a low risk of serious complications, comparable to that of pallidotomy. The main difference is the risk of infection and of electrodes breaking. Infection usually requires removing the electrode and stimulator. Electrode breakage requires surgery to remove the broken electrode. Other side effects depend on the brain area that is stimulated. For example, stimulation of the STN can cause dyskinesias; stimulation of the GPi induces muscular contractions or visual flashes in some people.

Bilateral stimulation of the GPi does not seem to have the same high rate of serious complications as bilateral pallidotomies, and published results suggest that the outcome is quite satisfactory. Patients with a unilateral pallidotomy can have good results using electrical stimulation on the other side, rather than risk bilateral pallidotomy.

## ►HIGH FREQUENCY STIMULATION VERSUS PALLIDOTOMY

No scientific study has as yet compared the two surgical procedures. A review of the medical literature suggests that some of the disadvantages of high frequency electrical stimulation compared to pallidotomy are:

- Two surgical procedures are needed: one to place the electrode and one to place the stimulator;
- The stimulator requires multiple adjustments involving many office visits;
- Battery changes are needed;
- Infection and electrode breakage can occur.

Some of the advantages of high frequency stimulation compared to pallidotomy are:

- The procedure is reversible and patients can turn the stimulation off whenever they choose to;
- Reversibility also means that patients can stop using their stimulator if a new treatment is discovered that is even better than high frequency stimulation or pallidotomy;
- The level of stimulation can be tailored to the patient's response;
- It is easy to test whether someone will respond to the procedure or not. If there is no response, all that needs to be done is to pull out the electrodes and try something else; and
- Bilateral stimulation is usually not a problem.

## ▶ SUMMARY

Neurosurgery for Parkinson's disease should in many ways still be considered experimental. Pallidotomy can relieve some of the symptoms that plague late-stage patients, but it is not a panacea. High frequency electrical stimulation seems to provide the same type of benefit. It has the advantage of being reversible but the disadvantage of requiring two surgical procedures instead of one, as well as more office visits. Many scientists hope and believe that by the time these techniques are perfected, the cause of Parkinson's disease will have been identified and a cure discovered, making neurosurgery obsolete.

# 5

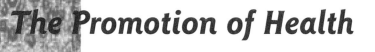

# The Promotion of Health

How can someone who has a chronic medical condition like Parkinson's disease also be healthy? The answer is to choose behaviors that promote health, defined as the optimal level of function and well-being. Despite the limitations that may be imposed by Parkinson's disease, one's overall physical and emotional capacity can be nurtured, and improvement achieved within realistic goals. This broad and positive approach to health can be conceptualized as "wellness," with emphasis placed on those areas within our control and on opportunities to make thoughtful and informed choices that will enhance our function, attitudes, and general sense of well-being.

## ▶ EXERCISE

Exercise is important for everyone, and people with Parkinson's disease should exercise regularly and with moderation. Too often, they stop exercising because stiff muscles and slowed movement (bradykinesia) make physical activity more difficult. Although no amount of exercise can modify the basic neurologic disease, those who continue to keep physically active do better in the long run than those who do not.

A few years ago a small, but rigorously conducted study confirmed the importance of regular exercise. The test subjects received two-hour rehabilitation sessions three times a week for four weeks, alternating with a control period without rehabilitation. The two periods were separated by six months and were assigned randomly to each patient (some received physical rehabilitation first and others received no rehabilitation first). To avoid examiner bias, patients were rated by an examiner who did not know the period in which they were participating. Ratings were done using a standardized battery of tests that evaluate motor functions, activities of daily living, and mental functions. Participants in the study were rated immediately before and after each period.

Scores of activities of daily living and motor function improved substantially after completion of the intensive rehabilitation program. These improvements were highly statistically significant. No change was observed in mental function scores. No significant improvement was found after the period without rehabilitation in any of the measures. This study clearly demonstrated the importance of regular physical therapy for people with Parkinson's disease.

Subsequent studies confirmed that exercise is beneficial for people with Parkinson's disease. Exercise helps improve motor function without an increase in medication. Many physicians are convinced that patients have better mobility using less medication when they exercise routinely

People with Parkinson's disease should work with their physicians, family members, and support groups to develop a weekly program of exercise and physical therapy to complement their medication schedule. A program of stretching, walking, and running is always beneficial, as is practicing skills used daily for a variety of tasks. A number of exercise routines are available for patients with Parkinson's disease, most of which are in the form of written instructions. Because many people find it easier to exercise with the assistance of a videotape, an exercise fitness tape titled "Sit and Be Fit" was specifically made for people with Parkinson's disease. It leads the viewer through a 20-minute exercise routine that consists of a series of gentle, slow movements designed to stretch and strengthen muscles and joints.

## ▶ DIET

Little is known about any possible relationship between diet and Parkinson's disease. Because most investigators agree that diet alone will never be sufficient to cure the disease, it is not considered a high research priority.

It is essential that people with Parkinson's disease eat well. Everyone needs a balanced diet, but people with any medical problem need it more than most because they cannot afford to add malnutrition to the burden of their disease. A well-balanced diet includes plenty of fresh fruits and vegetables, enough protein, and roughage. People often take supplements to increase their dietary intake of vitamins, but many nutritionists do not believe that this is an adequate substitute for a diet rich in fruits and vegetables.

## ▶ DIETARY CONSIDERATIONS SPECIFIC TO PARKINSON'S DISEASE

Meals with a high protein content can interfere with the absorption of levodopa (see Chapter 2), and low-protein diets significantly decrease the dose of levodopa that patients need. Some also find low-protein diets helpful to control "off" periods. Several low-protein food products have been recently made available commercially that claim to provide a nutritionally well-balanced diet that helps patients with motor fluctuations. However, many people soon tire of these diets. Most physicians prefer that their patients follow a normal diet rather than a low-protein diet, and that the dose of levodopa be adjusted to their needs. It is crucial to follow the chosen diet, since sudden changes will result in being either under- or overdosed. Whatever diet is chosen, meals should be eaten at regular times and gastronomic excesses should be avoided. Alcohol is acceptable in moderation.

Nausea and loss of appetite are common in Parkinson's disease and can lead to malnutrition because patients simply do not want to eat. These symptoms seem to be due in part to the disease itself and in part to antiparkinsonian medication. Treatments for these problems are described in Chapter 3. Having smaller but more frequent meals can help decrease nausea and loss of appetite. Snacking at 11:00 A.M. and again at 4:00 P.M. helps patients get a normal daily intake of food while eating less at lunch and dinner.

Another reason why people with Parkinson's disease eat too little is that they must eat very slowly due to a decreased rate of swallowing (see Chapter 3). Liquids and solids are difficult to swallow; soft foods are usually easiest. Hurrying only makes things worse. Patients should accept the situation and eat slowly and steadily. Eating slowly should not be an excuse to eat less. Antiparkinsonian medication often improves swallowing.

Constipation is common in Parkinson's disease. It also is both a consequence of the disease itself and a side effect of certain antiparkinsonian medications. To minimize constipation without taking laxatives, patients should regularly eat foods that contain natural laxatives (such as prunes or figs) and should drink four to eight glasses of water a day even if they are not thirsty.

Several lines of evidence point toward the involvement of free radicals in the genesis of Parkinson's disease. People with the disease therefore ask whether they should take supplements of vitamins, such as vitamins C or E, which "scavenge" free radicals. People with Parkinson's disease are no more susceptible to vitamin deficiencies than the general population, and a normal diet usually contains enough of these vitamins. It is probably a good idea to take a multivitamin pill per day as insurance against poor eating habits. Vitamins cannot cure Parkinson's disease, and some, like vitamin E, hardly enter the brain.

In conclusion, people with Parkinson's disease should eat normally and follow a well-balanced diet. They should take the time and trouble to eat enough. Vitamin supplements in normal doses may be of benefit and seem to do no harm. People with Parkinson's disease should not have unreasonable hopes about diet, as it seems unlikely that the cause or the treatment of the disease resides in nutrition.

## ▶PATIENT EDUCATION AND HEALTH PROMOTION

A program of patient education and health promotion can be an effective adjunct to the management of Parkinson's disease. This type of program is inexpensive, reduces medical costs, and improves the value of therapy, as was demonstrated in a six-month randomized, controlled clinical trial involving 290 patients with Parkinson's disease. Half the patients were enlisted in the patient education and health promotion program, whereas the other half were not. All participants were sent a health promotion program called **PROPATH** via mail and questionnaires requesting information on symptoms at time of entry into the study and at two, four, and six months. Those in the education and health promotion group were also provided with a computer-generated individualized recommendation letter and a report that summarized their progress over time, along with pamphlets and educational materials detailing information on individualized exercise recommendations, diet, compliance, control of side effects, and coping with reported problems. With each two-month cycle, the physicians of the "educated" group were sent a summary report listing the recommendations given to their patient(s) and suggestions for physician consideration. Six months after the start of the study, both groups were administered a quality-of-life test battery that assessed self-efficacy; an additional questionnaire was completed by the spouse or caregiver of each patient to assess the level of stress experienced by that person.

At the beginning of the study, both groups were comparable for duration and severity of disease, side-effect profiles, exercise regimens, and disease progression rates. Patients in the "educated" group showed statistically significant improvement and a significant decrease in visits to the doctor, while those in the "noneducated" group worsened significantly. At the end of the six-month study, the "educated" group fared better on most of the variables assessed. Doses of levodopa and bromocriptine were lower, as was utilization of medical services. Self-efficacy beliefs about controlling symptoms and managing the disease were better. Spousal reports also favored this group, although not to a statistically significant degree. At the end of the trial, patients in the "noneducated" group were offered the entire program. In summary, the program stabilized disease progression, improved exercise frequency and health confidence, decreased the need for medication, and decreased physician office visits.

# Section

# II

## IMPROVING THE
## MANAGEMENT OF
## PARKINSON'S DISEASE

# 6

# Research on Parkinson's Disease: An Overview

Thirty years after its discovery, levodopa is still the best treatment for Parkinson's disease, but there is a substantial need for improvement.

- Treatments are needed to improve the treatment of both the primary symptoms of Parkinson's disease and its long-term complications and side effects. It would be helpful if patients needed to take medication only once or twice a day to minimize peak-dose side effects and end-of-dose deterioration. Treatments are especially needed for the late-stage complications that tend to appear after a number of years of treatment and do not respond to levodopa.
- Most importantly, patients are waiting for a treatment that will stop the loss of nerve cells that underlies Parkinson's disease. The best way to find a cure is to discover the cause of the disease, and research on possible causes is progressing rapidly.
- If nerve cell loss cannot be prevented, another way to restore motor function might be to replace missing nerve cells.

Section II of this book examines the search for new treatments of Parkinson's disease and is organized according to this list of needs. Chapters 8 and 9 deal with the search for long-acting treatments. Chapter 10 describes ongoing research on the cause of late-stage motor complications and analyzes how that research could lead to treatments for symptoms that do not respond well to levodopa. Chapters 11, 12, and 13 summarize current research on the cause of Parkinson's disease and delineate the types of treatments that might as a consequence help slow or stop progression. Chapter 14 outlines ongoing efforts to improve neuronal transplantation and replacement of missing cells.

## ►ANIMAL MODELS OF PARKINSON'S DISEASE

Animal research is the basis for the development of all medical therapies, and animal models that mimic the human disease are essential to finding new treatments. Two main models of Parkinson's disease are used to test new drugs and other therapies. Both models use toxins that selectively destroy substantia nigra nerve cells. Six-hydroxydopamine is used in rats, while MPTP is used in monkeys. These models are discussed here and will be referred to constantly in succeeding chapters.

### The 6-Hydroxydopamine Model

In this model, the toxin 6-hydroxydopamine is injected into the substantia nigra of rats, causing rapid and severe degeneration of dopamine nerve cells. The resulting lesion reproduces the brain lesion that characterizes Parkinson's disease. The major difference is that the lesion is "fixed," and there is no continuing progressive loss of neurons. In the rat model, 6-hydroxydopamine is usually injected only on one side of the brain, mimicking hemiparkinsonism. In large doses, the toxin typically causes degeneration of more than 95 percent of the dopamine neurons, which is comparable to advanced Parkinson's disease. Smaller doses can also be used, and the resulting loss of a smaller percentage of neurons mimics an earlier stage of Parkinson's disease. Thus, researchers can choose which stage of the disease they wish to study for any given experiment.

Rats with substantia nigra lesions do not have the same symptoms as people. Instead of obvious tremor or rigidity (stiffness), they show "postural asymmetry," and when given levodopa they turn in circles toward the side opposite to the side where the lesion was placed. The time during which the rats exhibit this turning behavior reflects the duration of action of levodopa. In an experimental situation, changes in the duration of turning behavior provide a measurement of the effectiveness of the therapy being studied.

The process by which 6-hydroxydopamine destroys substantia nigra nerve cells involves the release of substantial amounts of free radicals. As discussed in Chapter 13, it is believed that excessive free radicals may contribute to the development of Parkinson's disease in humans.

## The MPTP Model

In 1977 a college student suddenly developed a severe form of what appeared to be Parkinson's disease. When he arrived at the emergency room, his hands were trembling, his face was immobile and expressionless, his body movements were slow, and he could not talk. A neurologic consultant diagnosed parkinsonism but was puzzled by the rapidity with which the disease had developed. The patient was treated with levodopa, and within days he was walking and able to provide information about what had happened. He was a drug addict and over the previous months had been injecting himself with a homemade heroin substitute, a synthetic compound called MPPP (1-methyl-4-phenyl-1,2,3,6-tetrahydropyridine), which is chemically related to Demerol. Making this substance is simple, but relatively minor errors in procedure lead to the formation of the related compound MPTP (N-methylphenyl tetrahydropyridine). When chemists at the National Institutes of Health (NIH) followed the patient's "recipe," they found that indeed the final product was a mixture of these substances. This mixture was not very toxic in rats but destroyed substantia nigra nerve cells in monkeys. Researchers concluded that the homemade MPPP/MPTP mixture could have caused parkinsonism in this patient. When he died a year later following an overdose of cocaine, an autopsy confirmed that he had lost most of his substantia nigra nerve cells.

A few years later, "designer drug" chemists in California began supplying their customers with "synthetic heroin." They also were trying to make pure MPPP but instead made a mixture of MPPP and MPTP. Before long, drug addicts were arriving at emergency rooms with what appeared to be sudden-onset severe Parkinson's disease; they improved dramatically with levodopa. The neurologist in California who saw these patients also linked the disease to the "synthetic heroin," and analysis of a sample of the illicit drug showed it to contain MPTP. When administered to monkeys, this MPTP caused lesions of substantia nigra nerve cells that were similar to those of Parkinson's disease. The monkeys also exhibited motor symptoms that closely resemble those of Parkinson's disease.

The lesion can be reliably and consistently reproduced, giving researchers an excellent tool in which to study a variety of therapies designed to treat parkinsonian symptoms and prevent progress of the disease.

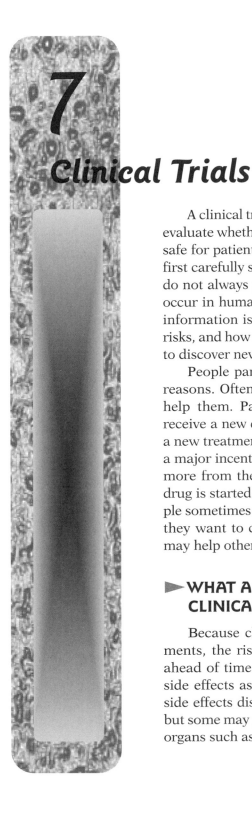

# 7

# *Clinical Trials*

A clinical trial is a scientific study conducted to evaluate whether a new treatment is beneficial and safe for patients with a specific disorder. A drug is first carefully studied in animals, but these studies do not always predict all the side effects that may occur in humans. During each clinical trial, more information is gained about a new treatment, its risks, and how effective it might be. It is impossible to discover new drugs without clinical trials.

People participate in clinical trials for many reasons. Often they hope the new treatment will help them. Participants are among the first to receive a new drug, sometimes many years before a new treatment is generally available. This can be a major incentive because it may be eight years or more from the time the first clinical trial with a drug is started to its approval for general use. People sometimes participate in clinical trials because they want to contribute to a research effort that may help others.

## ▶WHAT ARE THE RISKS OF CLINICAL TRIALS?

Because clinical trials investigate new treatments, the risks involved are not always known ahead of time. New drugs can cause unexpected side effects as well as anticipated benefits. Most side effects disappear when treatment is stopped, but some may persist and involve damage to major organs such as the heart, lung, and kidneys.

It can be difficult to decide whether to participate in a clinical trial. The potential risks must be weighed carefully against the possible benefits. You should not forget that available treatments also cause side effects and may involve some risk. If you are thinking about entering a clinical trial but are worried or confused about the information you have been given concerning the drug or the trial, you should not hesitate to discuss the matter with your physician. Most people find it helpful to have a friend or a relative with them when the clinical trial and the new drug are explained. You have a right to understand all aspects of the trial; no question is foolish, and you should feel completely informed about your choices as well as the risks and benefits of the various treatments available. Finally, remember that you can always refuse to join a study and that you can always leave a clinical trial at any time.

## ▶QUESTIONS TO ASK WHEN CONSIDERING PARTICIPATING IN A CLINICAL TRIAL

Deciding whether or not to participate in a clinical trial can be difficult. You should make a point of learning as much as you can about both the trial and the drug before making a decision. You should decide that you want to participate only after you feel confident that you understand the possible risks and benefits. It can be helpful to make a list of questions before talking to the medical staff in charge of the study. The following are some questions you might consider asking:

- Has the drug previously been given to people with Parkinson's disease? If so, was it given at the same dose and for the same duration as in the proposed clinical trial? What were the side effects? Was the drug helpful?
- Given your particular health problems (for example, hypertension or stomach ulcer), would you be more likely to suffer from side effects with the new drug than other drugs?
- What is the objective of the proposed clinical trial?
- What does the proposed trial involve? How long will it last?
- Can you continue to take other treatments during the trial? If not, what are the risks and disadvantages of stopping other treatments?
- What tests will be done?
- Will part of the trial be conducted in hospital? How many visits to the clinic will there be? Who will pay for travel?
- What are the alternative treatments? How do they compare with the new drug? What are the possible advantages/disadvantages of taking the new drug instead of those currently available?

- Who is the sponsor? (NIH? private foundation? pharmaceutical company?)
- Will you need to incur any costs? If you develop a side effect during the trial and need treatment (including hospitalization), who will pay for it?
- At the end of the trial, will you be allowed to continue taking the new drug if it is found to be beneficial? If so, for how long?

It often helps to write down your questions ahead of time. During the office visit, you can read your questions and write down the answers.

## ▶ HOW ARE CLINICAL TRIALS PERFORMED?

There are many kinds of clinical trials, and they can cover many different aspects of Parkinson's disease. Some trials investigate slowing disease progression, while others are concerned with improving its symptoms. In most cases the "treatments" are drugs, but they can also be surgical procedures such as pallidotomy, special diets, or life-style. Some clinical trials are carried out only at one institution, while others take place in several facilities across the country. Some trials are funded by the pharmaceutical industry, whereas others are sponsored by NIH or private foundations.

There are two major types of clinical trial in Parkinson's disease. The first examines whether treatment improves the symptoms of the disease. This can usually be evaluated over short periods of time, such as four to eight weeks. The second type of clinical trial examines whether a drug slows progression. Such an effect can only be evaluated over a prolonged period of time, usually 12 to 18 months.

Although some clinical trials examine the effects of only one treatment, most compare the effect of one treatment to another. Some studies investigate more than two therapies, and some compare several doses of a drug to determine which is optimal. In these comparative studies, each treatment (or dose) is given to a different group of people. Some trials compare the effects of a new drug to a placebo (an inert substance sometimes referred to as a sugar pill), while others compare the new drug to one that is commercially available.

In some clinical trials, patients are exposed only to one treatment. For example, if a study compares Treatment A to Treatment B, one group receives Treatment A and the other receives treatment B. In other trials, one group of patients receives Treatment A followed by Treatment B, while another receives Treatment B followed by Treatment A. Patients usually prefer being offered a chance to receive all treatments, but this type of design is not always possible and depends on the objective of the study.

Most clinical trials are performed with new drugs that are not yet commercially available, but some are conducted to test new uses for older drugs. The DATATOP study examined whether a known drug like selegiline (Eldepryl®) could slow the progression of Parkinson's disease (see Chapter 2). Before the study, selegiline was used to prolong and smooth the effects of levodopa. Another example of old drugs being studied for new uses is the clinical trial that is ongoing to find out if early treatment with a controlled release formulation of levodopa (Sinemet CR®) will decrease the risk of late-stage complications.

## ►AVOIDING BIAS IN CLINICAL TRIALS

One way to avoid bias of the patient or of the physician from influencing the results of the study is randomization, with people selected by chance to be included in a given treatment group. An additional way to prevent bias is to conduct a "double-blind" clinical trial, in which neither the patient nor the physician knows which treatment the patient is receiving. Health authorities, such as the Food and Drug Administration (FDA) in the United States, require that the benefits of a drug be demonstrated in randomized and double-blind studies before the drug is made generally available.

## ►THE STAGES OF CLINICAL TRIALS

Drugs are extensively tested in the laboratory for possible toxicity or side effects before they are given to patients. Because laboratory studies cannot always predict exactly what a drug will do to people, they must be rigorously tested. Clinical trials for Parkinson's disease are normally carried out in four phases, each of which provides information that allows progression to the next phase.

### Phase I

The first phase of a clinical trial has two objectives: to find out if the new treatment has any unexpected side effects that might not have been detected in animals, and to determine whether the drug enters the bloodstream and how long it stays there in order to determine how often it should be given during each day.

This phase is usually done in young healthy subjects. There is an ongoing debate in the medical community about whether this is right. Some say that it is not ethical to expose healthy people to the risk of a new drug that cannot benefit them. Additionally, the side effects of drugs can be very different in healthy people and in those with a disease. Others say that it is not ethical to expose a patient who is already burdened and weakened by disease to the risk of additional problems.

When a drug is given for the first time to humans, the initial dose will be very low, usually one tenth of the dose expected to be beneficial. If the initial low dose does not cause problems, it is gradually and cautiously increased until side effects are observed. Vital functions are monitored frequently during these early studies. Blood tests are repeated frequently to make sure that the drug does not affect important organs such as the liver or the kidneys. Special tests (such as those for memory) are sometimes done to make sure that the drug does not affect these functions. Finally, the blood levels of the new drug are carefully monitored.

The next phase of clinical trials begins only if the results of the first phase of clinical trials show that:

- Side effects (if any) are acceptable at the doses that are considered to be beneficial in patients; and
- The drug enters the bloodstream and remains there for a sufficiently long period.

### Phase II

The second phase of clinical trials tests whether the drug benefits patients and determines the optimal dose. Increasing the dose usually increases both benefits and side effects, so the "best" dose is determined by balancing beneficial effects against unwanted side effects. The new drug is usually compared to a placebo in this phase of testing. If the drug is shown to both benefit patients and have acceptable side effects, the third phase of clinical trials is begun.

### Phase III

The third phase compares the new drug at its best dose to already available drugs to determine whether the new treatment is better than available therapies. Examples of what can make a drug "better" are:

- The drug is more beneficial;
- It is as beneficial as an older treatment but has fewer side effects;
- It can be taken at a lower frequency than existing medications.

During this phase, the new drug is compared to available treatments in large studies that involve several hundred patients, usually in many centers.

At the same time these studies are being conducted, smaller studies are carried out in patients with special problems, such as liver or kidney disease, to accurately assess any special risks of the drug. Small studies are also carried out to determine how the drug interacts with frequently prescribed medications, such as drugs for high blood pressure or anti-ulcer medications.

If the third phase of clinical testing confirms that the drug is beneficial and safe, a New Drug Application (NDA) is submitted to the FDA (or similar agencies in other countries) to obtain permission to put it on the market.

### Phase IV

Clinical trials continue once a new drug is on the market, both to confirm previous results and to obtain more information about side effects, some of which may be rare and therefore detected only after large numbers of people are taking the drug. Phase IV studies can involve thousands of patients.

## ►CLINICAL TRIALS TAKE MANY YEARS

The first phase of clinical trials usually involves 50 to 100 subjects and lasts from 6 months to a year; the second phase typically involves 200 to 400 patients and lasts approximately 3 years; and the third phase involves at least 1,000 patients and lasts 3 to 5 years. Finally, it often takes 2 to 3 years for the NDA to be approved. Thus, a new drug is typically made generally available 10 to 12 years after the first clinical trials begin.

## ►PROTECTION OF PATIENTS IN CLINICAL TRIALS

Clinical trials are carried out according to strict rules that guarantee maximum safety for participants. For each clinical trial, there is a *protocol*, a treatment plan that describes exactly what types of patients will participate in the trial, what procedures will be done, and when they will be done. This protocol is reviewed by an Institutional Review Board (IRB) at the institution where the clinical trial will take place. IRBs are intended to protect patients. They include scientists, physicians, clergy, and other people from the community. The IRB reviews the protocol to ascertain that it is well-designed and makes scientific sense, checks that the doses used are properly selected and that the risks are reasonable in relation to the potential benefits, and examines the information that is given to the patient in the Informed Consent Form to make sure it is honest and complete. In addition to the IRB review, protocols are usually carefully reviewed by the institutions where the studies are being conducted for medical ethics, patient safety, and scientific merit.

Once a clinical trial starts, safety results should be reviewed on an ongoing basis to determine whether any unforeseen side effect is occurring that substantially increases the risk to participants. Whenever possible, results should be periodically reviewed by a safety committee made up of physicians and scientists who are not involved in the trial. A safety committee may recommend stopping a clinical trial or putting it on hold until a particular result has been investigated.

## ►INFORMED CONSENT

Before joining a clinical trial, patients must give informed consent. Doctors and nurses provide information so that they can understand the new treatment and what is involved in participating in the trial. Potential benefits and risks are carefully explained so that patients can decide freely whether they want to join the trial. They are also given an Informed Consent Form that describes what is known about the drug and what is involved in the clinical trial (for example, what types of procedures and how many office visits are involved). Patients should read this document carefully and ask any questions they may have. They should sign the form only when they are fully informed and agree to take part in the study; they should then be given a copy for their records. Signing an Informed Consent Form does not bind a patient to stay in a study. Informed consent continues throughout the trial; participants are informed about any new finding that could affect their willingness to continue to participate in the study. Patients are always free to refuse to participate in a study, even after they have signed the Informed Consent Form.

## ►HOW CAN I FIND OUT WHICH CLINICAL TRIALS ARE ONGOING IN PARKINSON'S DISEASE?

Many people with Parkinson's disease are interested in participating in clinical trials, but they do not know how to obtain information on what trials are ongoing. In some diseases, such as Alzheimer's disease, AIDS, or cancer, lists of ongoing clinical trials are made available to patients. For each ongoing study, such lists usually give a short description of the drug being evaluated, the type of patient who is eligible for the trial, the design of the study, the clinical centers where the study is being conducted, the name and telephone number of the contact person, and information about the sponsor. Patients and their physicians can study these lists and decide in which trials they are most interested. A similar system does not exist for Parkinson's disease. Patient voluntary associations are usually a good source of information. The newsletter *Parkinson's Disease Update* often announces studies that are about to begin. The Experimental Therapeutics Branch (ETB) of the National Institute of Neurological Disorders and Stroke (NINDS) in Bethesda, Maryland, frequently conducts early clinical trials in patients. The Parkinson Study Group (PSG) coordinates many clinical trials in Parkinson's disease. Both ETB and PSG can be contacted for information (see Resources).

# 8

# Treatments That Prolong the Effects of Levodopa

Nearly all drugs now used in the management of Parkinson's disease provide symptomatic treatment; they do not delay or prevent progression of the disease process. Levodopa, the active ingredient of Sinemet® and Madopar®, remains the best treatment for the disease, but there is need for improvement. Two major problems of levodopa therapy are its tendency to become less helpful in the later stages of the disease and its short duration of action. The latter means that multiple daily dosing is necessary, and that in turn causes patients to "swing on" and "swing off" medication several times throughout the day. This is not only a source of discomfort, but it may also cause or accelerate the onset of late-stage motor fluctuations and peak-dose dyskinesias. Not surprisingly, the quest for better symptomatic treatments of Parkinson's disease focuses mainly on the development of long-acting medications and treatments for late-stage complications.

Current research on longer-acting drugs concentrates on efforts to prolong the effects of levodopa and the search for long-acting dopamine agonists.

## ►TREATMENTS THAT PROLONG THE HALF-LIFE OF LEVODOPA

### Controlled-Release Formulations

Controlled-release formulations slowly release levodopa in the stomach and bowel. They increase its duration of action, allowing for smoother effects and less frequent daily dosing. Two such formulations are currently available, Sinemet CR® and Madopar HBS® (not available in the United States). A few research groups are looking for better controlled-release formulations, but none has yet emerged.

### Liquid Levodopa/Carbidopa

Drinking small amounts of liquid Sinemet® at frequent intervals seems to maintain steady levels of levodopa in the bloodstream, as described in Chapter 2.

### Prodrugs

A long-acting levodopa effect can also be obtained by using a "prodrug" to produce a slow release of levodopa into the bloodstream. This type of drug is taken orally and absorbed unchanged from the bowel into the bloodstream. Once in the bloodstream, it is metabolized and slowly releases levodopa over several hours. The levodopa prodrug LME (levodopa-methyl ester) has a longer duration of action and smoother effects than levodopa but a slower onset of action. A more recently discovered prodrug of levodopa, NB-355, extends the duration of action of levodopa and produces less severe dyskinesias.

### Combination of Levodopa with a Decarboxylase Inhibitor

A prodrug that slowly releases levodopa in the bloodstream must be combined with a decarboxylase (DC) inhibitor to minimize the formation of dopamine outside the brain, thus substantially reducing the side effects of levodopa, especially nausea and postural hypotension. Both carbidopa and benserazide block DC in the bloodstream but not in the brain; levodopa and carbidopa are combined in Sinemet®, and the combination of levodopa and benserazide is Madopar®.

The need to use a DC inhibitor with a levodopa prodrug is a major deterrent to conducting research in this area. There are no commercially available DC inhibitors; carbidopa and benserazide are only sold combined with levodopa. If a pharmaceutical company were to develop a levodopa prodrug, they would have to discover and develop their own DC inhibitor, and those that do not enter the brain are not easy to find. Moreover, the need to associate two drugs (the prodrug and the DC inhibitor) would double the cost of development.

Some pharmaceutical companies are trying to make prodrugs that slowly release dopamine directly into the brain, instead of levodopa. The underlying concept is that the prodrug will be absorbed from the bowel into the bloodstream and will circulate unchanged and be taken up into the brain, where it will slowly release dopamine. No DC inhibitor would be needed with this type of prodrug, but none is yet ready for clinical testing.

### COMT Inhibitors

When DC inhibitors were associated with levodopa, researchers hoped that blocking DC would prolong the duration of action of levodopa and reduce side effects. This did not happen because another enzyme, catechol-ortho-methyl-transferase (COMT), degraded levodopa into 3-O-methyl-dopa (3-OMD; Figure 8-1).

Only about 1 percent of the levodopa taken orally reaches the brain because levodopa is degraded by COMT in the gut and a number of internal organs (Figure 8.2). Blocking COMT in the bowel and the liver should both prolong the effects of levodopa and allow its daily dose to be decreased.

The first drugs that blocked COMT, known as *COMT inhibitors*, were discovered more than 20 years ago, but they were toxic and their use was abandoned. Two well-tolerated COMT inhibitors are now available—entacapone and tolcapone.

Entacapone blocks COMT in the bowel and liver but not in the brain. When given together with Sinemet® or Madopar®, entacapone approximately doubles the duration of action of levodopa without increasing the

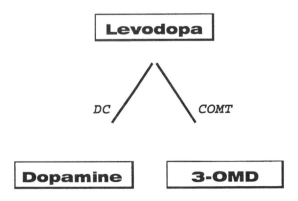

*Figure 8-1.* Levodopa is primarily degraded by two enzymes, a decarboxylase (DC) and a catechol-ortho-methyl-transferase (COMT).

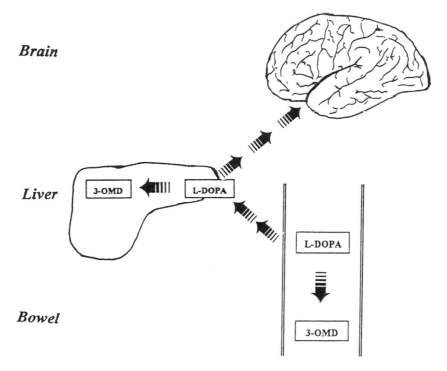

*Brain*

*Liver*

*Bowel*

*Figure 8.2.* COMT degrades levodopa in many places, but especially in the bowel, the liver, and the brain. In the brain, COMT also degrades dopamine (see Figure 8.3).

*severity* of dyskinesias. However, it does increase the *duration* of dyskinesias by prolonging the half-life of levodopa in the bloodstream.

Unlike entacapone, tolcapone blocks COMT in the brain as well as in the bowel and liver (Figure 8.3). Its effects are similar to those of entacapone when given together with Sinemet® or Madopar®, with an approximate doubling of the duration of action of levodopa and no increase in the severity of dyskinesias but an increase in their duration.

Both drugs are undergoing final clinical testing in Europe, the United States, and Japan and will probably be available commercially within a few years. One of the problems with both drugs is their short half-life. If they were long-acting, associating them with slow release preparations of levodopa such as Sinemet CR® might result in prolonged and smooth effects. The search for a long-acting COMT inhibitor is currently ongoing but no drug has yet emerged.

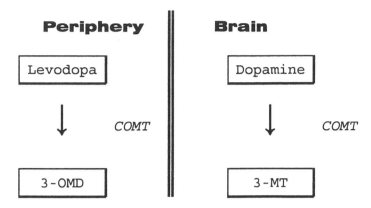

*Figure 8.3.* In the striatum, COMT degrades dopamine into 3-MT (3-methoxytyramine).

## ►GENETICALLY ENGINEERED CELLS TO STABILIZE THE RESPONSE TO LEVODOPA

Are there any other ways to obtain prolonged and stable levels of levodopa in the bloodstream? One way would be to engineer cells that continuously make and release levodopa, "pack" them in a capsule, and implant them under the skin. The capsules would permit the inward diffusion of nutrients and the outward diffusion of levodopa. Encapsulating the cells has two additional advantages: it protects the grafted cells from attack by the immune system, and it prevents their moving away from the implant site. As in the case of pro-drugs, this type of treatment would need to be associated with a DC inhibitor. Genetically engineered cells are now in the early stages of research, and many technical hurdles need to be overcome before they become available.

## ►TREATMENTS THAT STABILIZE DOPAMINE LEVELS IN THE BRAIN

Dopamine is degraded by several enzymes in the brain, one of which, monoamine oxidase type B (MAO-B), degrades dopamine into an inactive compound called *DOPAC*. Drugs such as selegiline that block MAO-B therefore increase the duration of action of dopamine. Clinical trials have shown that adding selegiline to levodopa prolongs its duration of action and smooths its effects in advanced stages of the disease. However, the emphasis with these compounds has thus far been placed on prevention of progression rather than on increasing the duration of action of levodopa.

Another approach to maintaining constant levels of dopamine in the striatum would be to transplant fetal cells or genetically engineered cells that continuously make and release dopamine. Several groups are actively trying to obtain such cells, but a great deal more research is needed before this type of technology can be safely used in people with Parkinson's disease.

## ►CONCLUSION

The quality of life of people with Parkinson's disease would be significantly improved if the duration of action of levodopa could be sufficiently prolonged. They would have fewer peak-dose side effects and would not have to worry about wearing-off. Today the duration of action of levodopa can at best be doubled, using either controlled-release preparations of levodopa or COMT inhibitors. Genetically engineered cells might allow for continuous and smooth production of levodopa over several weeks, but the technology is far from being commercially available. Another way to obtain prolonged and stable control of motor symptoms would be to find long-acting drugs that mimic the effects of dopamine. The search for this type of drug is described in Chapter 9.

# 9

# The Search for Long-Acting Dopamine Agonists

In Parkinson's disease the progressive loss of nerve cells from the substantia nigra causes the concentrations of dopamine in the striatum to slowly decrease. As a result, striatal dopamine receptors receive less stimulation, and this reduced stimulation causes the symptoms of the disease. Replacing the missing dopamine is the principle underlying levodopa therapy. A logical alternative would be to treat Parkinson's disease with drugs that directly stimulate dopamine receptors. Substances other than dopamine itself that bind to dopamine receptors and stimulates them, or "dopamine agonists," have many theoretical advantages compared to levodopa.

- Because they do not need to be stored in and released by substantia nigra neurons, they should continue to be beneficial even in late-stage disease when most nigral nerve cells are lost.
- They could be longer-acting than levodopa, and once or twice a day dosing is conceivable.
- If they were long-acting, they might prevent or delay the onset of late-stage motor complications such as wearing-off and peak-dose dyskinesias.

Apomorphine is the oldest known dopamine agonist. It is not active when taken orally but is nearly as effective as levodopa when infused intravenously. This supports the concept that levodopa therapy could be replaced by dopamine agonists.

The search for dopamine receptor stimulants that would be active when taken orally and continue to be active in advanced disease led to the discovery of bromocriptine (Parlodel®), pergolide (Permax®), and lisuride (Dopergine®, which is not available in the United States). These dopamine agonists are not as effective as levodopa and cannot replace it when taken alone. As a result, they are usually given in the early stages of the disease when patients do not yet need levodopa, or in combination with levodopa to enhance its effects in more advanced patients. The reason that existing dopamine agonists are not as helpful as levodopa is unknown, but recent discoveries about dopamine receptors suggest that it may be possible to develop agonists that work as well as levodopa. It would be fairly simple to make such compounds long-acting and thus overcome two of the problems of levodopa therapy—its reduced efficacy in advanced stages of the disease and the need for multiple dosing throughout the day.

## ▶NEW RECEPTORS FOR DOPAMINE

Only two dopamine receptors were known until recently, the D1 and the D2 types. Drugs that block D2 receptors, the *neuroleptics*, are used to treat mental illnesses such as schizophrenia. One of their major side effects is parkinsonism, which led to the belief that loss of D2 receptor stimulation causes the symptoms of Parkinson's disease. The search for dopamine agonists for Parkinson's disease therefore focused on the search for compounds that mainly stimulate this receptor. Two other dopamine receptors were recently discovered, the D3 and D4 types.

The D4 type is probably not involved since there are very few in the striatum, and parkinsonian symptoms are not seen in patients taking clozapine, which blocks the D4 receptor and is used to treat schizophrenia. The D3 receptor may be critical for the treatment of Parkinson's disease, and many believe that the beneficial effects of pramipexole, a new dopamine agonist, may be linked to its actions on the D3 receptor.

The ability of dopamine to reverse parkinsonian symptoms might conceivably be due mainly to its interaction with one receptor type, while side effects might be due to interaction with another. If that is true, it should be possible to discover drugs that reverse parkinsonian symptoms but have fewer side effects than levodopa because they do not stimulate the "side effect" receptor. The question then becomes which receptor to target. There is no consensus on this issue at present.

## ▶THE UNIQUE BINDING PROFILE OF DOPAMINE

Dopamine does not bind to all receptors in the same way. It binds most tightly (i.e., with the highest affinity) to D3 receptors, less to D2 receptors, and still somewhat less to D1 receptors. These differences in binding affinities constitute its "binding profile." Some scientists believe that a dopamine agonist should have the same binding profile as dopamine in order to work as well as levodopa. Currently available dopamine agonists have a binding profile somewhat different from that of dopamine, which may be why they are less effective than levodopa.

Dopamine binds with nearly equal strength to D1 and D2 receptors, and this equal strength profile may be the key to its beneficial effects. Apomorphine also binds with comparable strength to D1 and D2 receptors, which may be why it is the best agonist now available.

Dopamine stimulates all its receptors, but some agonists stimulate one receptor type and block another. For example, bromocriptine (Parlodel®) stimulates the D2 receptor but weakly blocks the D1 type.

## ▶D2 RECEPTOR AGONISTS

Bromocriptine (Parlodel®) is a D2 receptor agonist that has well-established antiparkinsonian effects, so there is no doubt that stimulation of this receptor type is beneficial. The fact that it does not work as well as levodopa suggests that stimulation of other receptor types may be necessary to obtain a maximally beneficial effect.

Drugs that stimulate the D2 receptor block the formation and secretion of prolactin by the pituitary gland and are beneficial in many conditions in which blood levels of this hormone are increased. Prolactin induces post-childbirth lactation, during which its concentrations increase significantly. D2 agonists block the increase in both prolactin and lactation; bromocriptine (Parlodel®) is often prescribed for this purpose. The effects of D2 agonists on prolactin are sometimes also used as a quick and reliable test to measure their duration of action. Long-acting D2 agonists would cause a prolonged suppression of prolactin.

Cabergoline is more potent and longer-acting than other agonists currently used to treat Parkinson's disease. It is available in Europe for the inhibition of normal post-partum lactation and for Parkinson's disease; it is not yet available in the United States. Clinical studies in the United States have shown that the drug is useful in patients treated with levodopa who experience motor fluctuations. Its once daily schedule and long-acting effects make the drug easier to take and provide greater control over fluctuations. Its most common side effects are dizziness, dry mouth, and orthostatic hypotension (a fall in blood pressure upon standing, which can cause dizziness). Cabergoline causes visual hallucinations in a small number of people.

Ropinerole is a D2 agonist that does not seem to interact at all with D1 receptors. The major problem is its short half-life and consequent short duration of action. Several hundred people with Parkinson's disease have been enrolled in clinical trials, and the drug seems to be useful both in early patients not yet treated with levodopa and as an adjunct to levodopa in more advanced patients. Side effects include nausea, vomiting, and orthostatic hypotension, which can be minimized by taking the drug with meals. Ropinirole may soon be available commercially.

Quinelorane is a long-acting D2 agonist that has been studied primarily for its effects on hyperprolactinemia (increased prolactin levels), sexual dysfunction, and infertility. To the best of our knowledge, this drug is not currently being tested in Parkinson's disease.

## ▶ D1 RECEPTOR AGONISTS

Some researchers believe that stimulation of the D1 receptor is essential to obtain strong antiparkinsonian effects, while others are convinced that D1 receptor agonists will only be marginally helpful.

There are several reasons to think that stimulation of the D1 receptor could be critical for the treatment of Parkinson's disease. For example, because it is the receptor for which dopamine has the lowest affinity and therefore requires the highest concentrations of dopamine to function, it might be the receptor type most affected in Parkinson's disease.

The D1 receptor is located "downstream" from D2 receptors, and it is now known that the D1 receptor acts like a "switch" that allows D2 receptor stimulation to be turned on. This interaction only occurs when substantia nigra neurons are intact, and lesions of these neurons "uncouple" the D1 from the D2 receptors. It is not known whether this process also occurs in Parkinson's disease. If it does, stimulation of D1 receptors might not be as beneficial as it is currently hoped.

Another subject of the debate concerning D1 receptor stimulants is the usefulness of stimulating *only* this receptor. Many studies suggest that D2 receptors must be stimulated to treat the symptoms of Parkinson's disease and that D1 receptor stimulation is needed only to turn on the D2 receptor. In this case, the best dopamine receptor stimulants for Parkinson's disease should be compounds that stimulate both. This is supported by clinical studies showing that pergolide (Permax®) is more effective than bromocriptine (Parlodel®). Bromocriptine is an antagonist at the D1 receptor, while pergolide is an agonist. Because pergolide is only a weak agonist at the D1 receptor, more potent agonists might be even more useful. Drugs that potently stimulate both receptor types are difficult to find; apomorphine is the best example.

Until recently there was no way to know if D1 receptor stimulants could be useful in Parkinson's disease because no drugs preferentially stimulated it. Several powerful D1 receptor stimulants were recently discovered and are currently being tested in humans. Dihydrexidine (DHX) behaves like a receptor stimulant in all laboratory experiments for D1 receptor functions in which it has been examined. Experiments in rats confirm that DHX is a full D1 agonist and does not have other activities. It completely reverses parkinsonian symptoms in MPTP monkeys. This suggests that stimulating only the D1 receptor might be enough to obtain beneficial effects in patients with Parkinson's disease. Unfortunately, DHX has a very short half-life and must be given intravenously because it is not absorbed from the bowel.

A-77636, a long-acting, highly selective D1 agonist, is a potent antiparkinsonian drug in rats and completely reverses parkinsonian symptoms in MPTP monkeys, in which it induces a more normal pattern of behavior than classic D2 agonists.

Several other D1 receptor agonists were recently shown to improve symptoms in parkinsonian animals. There may be at least two different D1 receptor subtypes, and stimulation of only one may be critical for the treatment of Parkinson's disease.

There are many reasons to be optimistic about the usefulness of D1 agonists, and researchers are waiting with great interest to know if these drugs are effective in people. Some predict a breakthrough. Whatever the result, studies of the effects of D1 agonists in patients with Parkinson's disease will provide useful clues as to how we should continue the search for better dopamine stimulants.

## ▶ AUTORECEPTOR BLOCKERS

The substantia nigra nerve terminals that release dopamine in the striatum carry "autoreceptors" (Figure 9.1) that interact with dopamine released in the synaptic cleft. These receptors are like sensors in that they can "feel" when dopamine has been released and tell the nerve terminal "levels of dopamine are high enough in the synaptic cleft; stop releasing it." If these

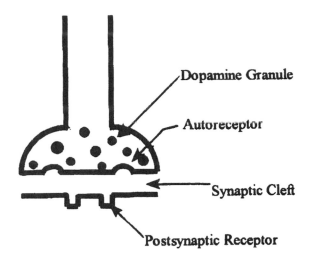

*Figure 9.1.* Schematic representation of autoreceptors at the dopamine synapse.

autoreceptors are blocked, substantia nigra neurons continuously release dopamine because they cannot sense its presence in the synaptic cleft.

Drugs that block dopamine autoreceptors could be useful in Parkinson's disease by increasing the release of dopamine. Autoreceptor blockers should be effective if stimulating receptors with the same binding profile as dopamine is critical, since they increase the levels of dopamine in the synaptic cleft. Drugs that block the autoreceptor could have a major advantage over levodopa because they can be made to be very long-acting. However, they would share with levodopa the disadvantage of losing efficacy with advancing disease as increasing numbers of nerve terminals are lost.

Pramipexole, a new drug that is reported to block dopamine autoreceptors, should increase the concentration of dopamine in the synapse. This drug also stimulates D2 and D3 receptors, and this combination of pre- and postsynaptic effects could make it very useful. Pramipexole has undergone final clinical testing in Europe and the United States and should soon be available commercially. Available data suggest that the drug could be of genuine value in the treatment of Parkinson's disease. In doses ranging from 0.1 mg to 5 mg daily, it seems to delay the need for levodopa and the development of dyskinesia, and some have suggested that perhaps it slows disease progression. End-of-dose wearing-off may also be reduced. Dizziness, nausea, vomiting, insomnia, and visual hallucinations were reported in some patients, but orthostatic hypotension was not a significant side effect.

## ▶APOMORPHINE: NEW WAYS TO ADMINISTER AN OLD DRUG

The beneficial effects of apomorphine have been known for more than a century. Early clinical trials confirmed that apomorphine has a potent, rapid, and predictable antiparkinsonian effect. It was not used clinically because of its side effects, especially vomiting, and because it could not be given by mouth. This situation has now changed because a drug called domperidone blocks the vomiting caused by apomorphine without blocking its antiparkinsonian effects, and as a result of the development of new drug delivery systems.

Most recent clinical studies of apomorphine have been conducted in Europe, where domperidone is available, but not in the United States. It is very useful in reversing parkinsonian symptoms during "off" periods. Some patients have been receiving apomorphine for more than five years without serious problems. It can either be injected intermittently using penjects (the type of syringe diabetics use to inject insulin) or it can be administered continuously by a portable pump. Intermittent administration is useful for people who can both anticipate the onset of their "off" periods and master the technique of self-injection. Clinical effects begin 5 to 15 minutes after injection and last for approximately one hour. Side effects consist mainly of nausea and drowsiness at the time the drug takes effect. A small number of people develop potentially serious side effects after the first dose of apomorphine, so treatment should be initiated in a hospital or clinic setting under direct medical observation. A few people may experience confusion and visual hallucinations, in which case treatment is halted. Some people also develop small, itchy lumps at the injection sites; this side effect ranges from minor discomfort to a major problem, so that apomorphine tends to be used only in advanced patients for whom other drugs are no longer useful. Some people who use injectable apomorphine particularly appreciate the confidence it gives them to know that their "off" periods can always be reversed.

Apomorphine can also be continuously infused using a portable pump, and it has been reported to maintain good mobility during the day, even in advanced patients. Results seem to be better when patients also receive intermittent oral levodopa, but apomorphine is very effective even without levodopa. Domperidone must be given to control nausea and vomiting for the first days or weeks of continuous infusion, but these side effects usually disappear after a few days.

The most frequent complication of continuous apomorphine infusion is the development of abdominal lumps at the site of the infusion and their occasionally becoming infected. This can usually be prevented by simple precautions such as changing needle sites daily, but some clinicians find this side effect to be troublesome enough to warrant using apomorphine only in patients who cannot be treated with other drugs.

To avoid the inconvenience of injections, other methods of drug delivery are being explored, including the intranasal route, sublingual tablets, or suppositories.

## ►SUMMARY AND CONCLUSIONS

Many drugs are being tested in the hope of improving the symptomatic treatment of Parkinson's disease. Research is moving in two main directions: prolonging the duration of action of levodopa, and the discovery of long-acting dopamine receptor stimulants that will work as well as or better than levodopa. Current results of both types of approaches look promising and may soon lead to drugs that will substantially improve the quality of life for many people.

# 10

# *Improving the Treatment of Late-Stage Complications*

Levodopa is less helpful in the later stages of Parkinson's disease due to motor complications such as end-of-dose wearing-off and peak-dose dyskinesias and the development of new symptoms that do not respond well to levodopa. These symptoms include speech and gait disturbances, postural instability, freezing episodes, levodopa-induced confusion, and depression. Several approaches to the treatment of late-stage complications have been identified and are being tested in animals, and some have already reached the stage of clinical testing.

The treatment of motor complications can focus on reducing their severity once they have begun (palliative therapy) or preventing their occurrence (preventive therapy), and some may do both. For example, stabilizing the levels of levodopa in the bloodstream helps to decrease the severity of motor fluctuations after they have started, but it may also delay the onset of late-stage motor complications.

## ►WEARING-OFF FLUCTUATIONS AND PEAK-DOSE DYSKINESIAS

End-of-dose deterioration or "wearing-off" is the most common and usually the first motor response complication. It is caused by a progressive shortening in the duration of effect of each dose of levodopa, so that patients need to take their medication increasingly more often. In advanced stages of the disease, the duration of effect may be so short that patients spend most of their time either "swinging on" or "swinging off" medication. Late-stage patients may also develop another form of motor response fluctuation called the on-off phenomenon, characterized by sudden, unpredictable switches between the untreated (parkinsonian) state and the overtreated (dyskinetic) stage.

Abnormal involuntary movements such as peak-dose dyskinesias can be extremely disabling. Levodopa does not induce dyskinesias in healthy people, except possibly at very high doses, but it *always* has the potential to induce dyskinesias in people with Parkinson's disease. In the early stages of the disease, peak-dose dyskinesias only occur with doses of levodopa that are much higher than that which improves parkinsonian symptoms. The dose that induces dyskinesias decreases steadily as the disease progresses, whereas that which improves symptoms does not change appreciably (Figure 10.1). As a result, the difference between the beneficial and dyskinetic doses of levodopa increasingly narrows. The beneficial and dyskinetic doses of levodopa become the same in some people with late-stage disease, who are then faced with the frustration of being able to have an "on" only when they develop dyskinesias.

## ▶BRAIN ABNORMALITIES THAT UNDERLIE MOTOR FLUCTUATIONS

The progressive shortening of the effects of levodopa and the lowering of the dyskinetic threshold were believed to result from the continuing slow and

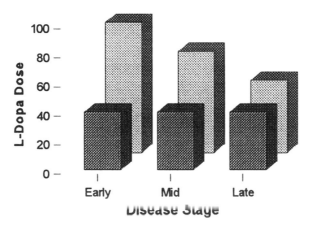

*Figure 10.1.* The beneficial dose of levodopa does not change appreciably as Parkinson's disease progresses, while that which causes peak-dose dyskinesias decreases steadily.

inexorable "burn-out" of dopamine neurons, and wearing-off fluctuations and peak-dose dyskinesias were considered inevitable with advanced Parkinson's disease. Recent research suggests that they in fact result, at least in part, from neuronal dysfunction caused by the short half-life of levodopa, and that some late-stage complications might be prevented or delayed by optimizing how levodopa is administered.

## ▶ DIFFERENT BRAIN CELLS SYNTHESIZE DOPAMINE IN EARLY AND ADVANCED DISEASE

In the early stages of Parkinson's disease, levodopa causes the remaining substantia nigra neurons to make more dopamine, thus compensating for lost neurons. As the number of neurons continues to decrease, the few that remain can no longer compensate. When the number of substantia nigra neurons falls to very low levels (5–10% of normal), the way in which the brain makes dopamine changes, and this change may at least partially underlie late-stage motor complications.

Orally administered levodopa is absorbed from the small bowel, enters the bloodstream, and eventually reaches the brain. In the early stages of the disease, it is taken up by substantia nigra nerve cells and converted into dopamine. This dopamine is stored in small vesicles in the neuronal terminals and released into the striatum at a relatively steady rate. This slow release accounts for the effectiveness of levodopa for several hours despite its rapid clearance from the bloodstream, and it is responsible for the smooth, complication-free response to levodopa experienced by people with early mild parkinsonism.

As more nigral nerve cells disappear, levodopa is no longer taken up primarily by dopamine neurons. Some is taken up and converted to dopamine by endothelial cells that surround the vast network of small blood vessels found throughout the brain and by glial cells that act mainly to support and protect neurons.

The contribution of these cells increases as the number of substantia nigra neurons decreases. Rather than storing dopamine and releasing it gradually, they release it immediately into the synaptic cleft. The lack of storage was thought to explain end-of-dose deterioration, and immediate release was considered to be the cause of peak-dose dyskinesias. More recent research suggests that the actual situation is more complex.

In one study of wearing-off, researchers infused levodopa intravenously, adjusting the dose to each patient's needs to optimally reduce parkinsonian symptoms. The infusion was maintained for several hours, was then abruptly stopped, and the time for parkinsonian symptoms to return was measured. As expected, the effects of levodopa infusion declined much faster in patients with advanced disease (because of lack of storage), which accounts for the wearing-off phenomenon in late-stage patients.

The same test then was performed with intravenous apomorphine, which directly stimulates dopamine receptors. Because apomorphine does not need to be converted to an active substance by substantia nigra neurons, its effects are independent of the number of surviving neurons. Wearing-off therefore should not be observed with apomorphine if it is due to lack of storage. Surprisingly, however, the effect of apomorphine declined faster after abrupt withdrawal in patients with advanced disease. Wearing-off therefore could not be attributed solely to a lack of storage.

Researchers then examined the mechanisms underlying levodopa-induced dyskinesias. The basis of these side effects was originally thought to be simple. Because dopamine is not stored in nerve terminals with advancing disease, its levels in the synaptic cleft are high immediately after each dose of levodopa, and these high post-dose concentrations of dopamine trigger dyskinesias (explaining why they are called peak-dose dyskinesias). The cause of this side effect was found to be more complex.

A systematic study of peak-dose dyskinesias using intravenous levodopa confirmed the well-known finding that the threshold dyskinetic dose of levodopa slowly decreases with advancing disease. The same study was repeated with intravenous apomorphine, whose peak concentrations in the synaptic cleft are the same in early- and late-stage disease. If dyskinesias were related *only* to peak concentrations in the synaptic cleft, the dose of apomorphine that causes them should be the same in early- and late-stage disease. Surprisingly, the pattern of response to apomorphine was similar to that for levodopa: the dyskinetic threshold was lower in patients with advanced disease. The increased severity and frequency of peak-dose dyskinesias in patients with advancing disease could not be explained solely by increased peak concentrations of dopamine in the synaptic cleft. As with wearing-off, something more must be involved.

## ►PARKINSONIAN RATS HAVE WEARING-OFF

Researchers then turned to the rat model of advanced Parkinson's disease to study end-of-dose wearing-off. When lesioned rats were treated twice a day with levodopa, the duration of the effect of each dose decreased by about 25 percent after three weeks of treatment; in other words, the rats were experiencing wearing-off. This could not be explained by a progressive loss of dopamine neurons since the rat lesions do not progress. Wearing-off could not therefore be due to continued loss of dopamine neurons, confirming the conclusion of the apomorphine tests in patients.

Animals whose lesions mimicked an earlier stage of Parkinson's disease did not develop wearing-off in the same test situation, analogous to the lack of wearing-off seen in the early stages of Parkinson's disease. Taken together, these results demonstrated that wearing-off only occurs when a relatively high proportion of substantia nigra dopamine neurons are lost and that it is at least partly due to a mechanism that does not involve the loss of substantia nigra nerve cells.

## ▶ WEARING-OFF IS CAUSED BY INTERMITTENT LEVODOPA TREATMENT

In further experiments, rats whose lesions mimicked advanced disease received steady state infusions of levodopa for three weeks, the total daily dose being the same as with intermittent therapy. Wearing-off was not observed when the duration of response to a single dose of levodopa was measured before and after the three-week infusion, showing that wearing-off is a result of relatively long-term exposure to *intermittent* levodopa therapy.

To examine whether this surprising finding could also be observed in parkinsonian patients, researchers measured the duration of response to levodopa after standard intermittent levodopa therapy and after a ten-day round-the-clock intravenous infusion. The duration of response was the same after both treatments in early-stage patients but was longer in late-stage patients after a ten-day intravenous infusion than after intermittent therapy. Continuous levodopa infusions thus improved its effectiveness in late-stage patients and caused them to have less wearing-off.

Taken together, the findings can be summarized as follows. In rats, long-term continuous levodopa infusion does not lead to the wearing-off or other motor response complications seen with intermittent therapy. We do not know if early treatment with levodopa infusions would prevent the occurrence of wearing-off or other motor response complications in people with Parkinson's disease. However, the observation that continuous levodopa infusions in patients who already experience wearing-off can decrease its severity suggests that infusion early in the disease might prevent or at least delay the development of this motor fluctuation. Continuous levodopa infusions are not feasible for practical reasons, but equivalent therapies may be possible.

A clinical study is currently ongoing to see if using Sinemet CR® in patients with early Parkinson's disease will delay the onset of late-stage motor complications. An alternative to the use of drugs that prolong and stabilize the half-life of levodopa is the use of long-acting dopamine agonists. The problem with this type of drug is to find one that works as well as levodopa.

## ▶ CONTINUOUS LEVODOPA THERAPY IS BENEFICIAL FOR PEAK-DOSE DYSKINESIAS

Researchers postulated that, as with wearing-off, the lower dyskinetic threshold in the late stages of Parkinson's disease could be reversed by continuous levodopa therapy. A clear-cut improvement of the dyskinetic threshold was obtained in late-stage patients treated with continuous, round-the-clock infusion of levodopa for eight to ten days, although it did not return to the levels usually seen in early-stage patients. More prolonged infusions are not possible because levodopa is acidic and harmful to the veins, which makes it difficult to determine whether the dyskinetic threshold might be even further improved with more extended infusion. Lisuride is a drug that directly stimulates dopamine receptors and is fairly well tolerated by the intravenous route. Infusion with this drug for three months resulted in substantial improvement of the dyskinetic threshold over that seen with 10-day levodopa infusion.

The motor fluctuations and dyskinesias that complicate the treatment of advanced Parkinson's disease thus seem to be at least partly due to intermittent levodopa therapy and can be partially reversed by treatments that provide continuous dopamine replacement.

Since the only difference between intermittent treatment and continuous infusion is that brain levels of levodopa and dopamine oscillate with intermittent treatment, two factors appear to be necessary for wearing-off or peak-dose dyskinesias to occur: a severe loss of dopamine neurons *combined with* chronic intermittent levodopa therapy.

The explanation for why both factors are needed would seem to be related to the involvement of glial and endothelial cells in the production of dopamine in late-stage disease, with their intermittent "dumping" of large amounts of dopamine onto its receptors, which normally are exposed to fairly constant levels of dopamine.

## ▶ DOPAMINE RECEPTORS AND INTERMITTENT LEVODOPA THERAPY

When dopamine is released into the synapse, it binds to receptors on the "postsynaptic" side, initiating a cascade of events that leads to its functional effects (Figure 10.2).

One explanation of how oscillating concentrations of dopamine could aggravate wearing-off is that dopamine receptors are built to deal with stable levels of dopamine and that oscillating levels might either decrease their number or damage them. Little if any change in the actual number of recep-

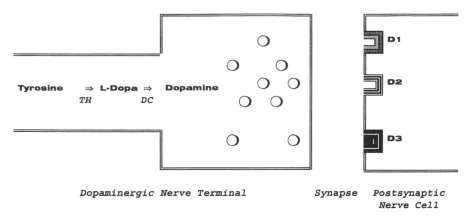

Figure 10.2. Schematic representation of a dopamine synapse. Not all nerve cells carry all three dopamine receptors.

tors was found in lesioned rats before and after three weeks of intermittent levodopa therapy.

When rats mimicking late-stage parkinsonism were tested with selective agonists before and after three weeks of intermittent levodopa therapy, they showed end-of-dose wearing-off and their response to a D1 selective agonist was greatly reduced. In contrast, their response to a D2 agonist was markedly enhanced, indicating that wearing-off is associated with an imbalance between the cascades of events triggered by the two types of receptors. The parkinsonian rats showing wearing-off had a "shut-down" of the neuronal system that is under D1 influence, so that most of dopamine's effects on the striatum were funneled through neurons carrying the D2 receptor.

The same experiment was then repeated with levodopa administered continuously via a pump. Rats mimicking late-stage disease were tested with selective D1 or D2 agonists before and after three weeks of therapy. The response to both agonists was the same before and after therapy, demonstrating that down-regulation of the D1-mediated response and up-regulation of the D2-mediated response do not occur when wearing-off does not occur.

Additional data to support the concept that wearing-off is linked to decreased D1- and increased D2-mediated responses were obtained in a situation in which intermittent treatment with levodopa does not produce wearing-off. Rats with only a partial lesion of the substantia nigra, resembling early parkinsonian patients, were tested with selective D1 or D2 agonists before and after chronic levodopa intermittent treatment. None developed wearing-off, and their responses to selective D1 or D2 agonists were no different before and after treatment. Once more, in a situation in which wearing-off did not occur, neither did shut-down of the D1-mediated response occur.

These results suggest that motor fluctuations such as wearing-off are due to an imbalance between striatal output pathways that are influenced by D1 and by D2 receptors. Recent data suggest that in parkinsonian patients, as in parkinsonian rats, most of the shortening in the response to levodopa reflects changes occurring in striatal neurons that receive dopaminergic terminals. This conclusion was reached by comparing the amount of shortening in the response to levodopa (whose action depends in part on the presence of dopamine terminals) to the amount of shortening in the response to apomorphine (which acts independently of dopamine terminals) in patients at various stages of the disease. These comparisons indicate that wearing-off is mainly due to secondary striatal changes that are a consequence of the unnatural intermittent interaction of dopamine with its receptors. It remains to be demonstrated that these secondary striatal changes in humans consist of reciprocal alterations in D1- and D2-mediated responses, as suggested by the animal experiments.

Just what are the pathways whose function is so profoundly influenced by chronic intermittent levodopa treatment?

## ▶ THE GLOBUS PALLIDUM AND LATE-STAGE COMPLICATIONS

Figure 10.3 is a greatly simplified representation of the neuronal circuits whose function is significantly modified by chronic, intermittent levodopa treatment.

As shown in Figure 10.3, there are two major pathways from the striatum to the internal segment of the globus pallidum (GPi). One is direct and involves neurons that carry mainly D1 receptors. A second pathway, which carries mainly D2 receptors, goes to the GPi indirectly via the GPe and the STN. Additionally, the cortex sends messages to the striatum and the STN and receives messages from the GPi via the VL. Smooth and easy movement is one of the results of the integration of these messages from different brain areas.

Under normal circumstances, dopamine release in the striatum causes a decrease in the activity of STN and GPi. Both are abnormally activated in Parkinson's disease, and many of the symptoms of the disease are now attributed to the heightened activity of the GPi, which acts like a "brake" on motor activity. Movement is slow and difficult to initiate for people with Parkinson's disease. Shut-down of the D1 pathway probably increases the activity of the GPi,

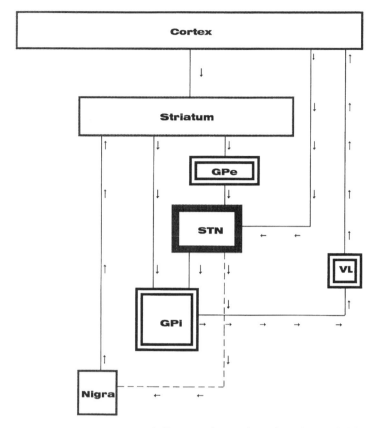

*Figure 10.3*. Schematic representation of efferent pathways from the striatum. GPi: internal segment globus pallidum; GPe: external segment globus pallidum; STN: subthalamic nucleus; VL: ventrolateral nucleus of thalamus.

explaining the appearance of late-stage motor complications. Drugs that stimulate the D1 receptor might help in the treatment of late-stage motor complications. Several D1 agonists are currently in the early stages of development.

Is it possible to release the GPi brake on motor activity? Although it has limitations, pallidotomy partially destroys the brake and is helpful in managing a number of the symptoms of the disease, especially levodopa-induced dyskinesias.

Most people would prefer to take medication rather than to undergo surgery. Glutamate antagonists that block the NMDA receptor in the striatum decrease the activity of the GPi and could possibly replace pallidotomy. However, glutamate antagonists have many side effects and are therefore poorly tolerated. Recent research suggests that it may be possible to discover glutamate antagonists that have minimal side effects.

## ►NEUROTRANSMITTERS IN THE DIRECT AND INDIRECT PATHWAYS

Another way to modulate the activity of the GPi may be to act on other neurotransmitter systems used by the direct and indirect pathways. All neurons use neurotransmitters to communicate with one another, and some use two or more at the same time (like some safes need more than one key); these neurotransmitters are "co-localized." The direct pathway from the striatum to the GPi uses the neurotransmitter GABA co-localized with dynorphin, substance P, and neurotensin. The indirect pathway from striatum to GPe uses GABA co-localized with enkephalin and neurotensin.

These neurotransmitters were measured in parkinsonian rats whose lesions mimicked late-stage disease. The results are summarized in Table 10.1.

**Table 10.1** *Effects of Nigral Lesions on Striatal Neurotransmitters in Rats*

| | Substantia Nigra Lesion | | |
| --- | --- | --- | --- |
| Neurotransmitter | No Treatment | Intermittent Levodopa | Continuous Levodopa |
| Enkephalin | ↑ | ↑ | Normal |
| Neurotensin | ↑ | ↑↑ | Normal |
| Dynorphin | N I | ↑↑ | Normal |

Loss of dopamine neurons increases striatal enkephalin and neurotensin levels, and intermittent levodopa treatment induces a massive increase in both dynorphin and neurotensin; this increase does not occur with continuous infusion. Since intermittent levodopa treatment causes late-stage complications in animals but continuous infusion does not, these complications probably are linked to the increase in dynorphin or neurotensin, or both. Therefore, another approach to the treatment of late-stage complications is to block the effects of either dynorphin or neurotensin. To date, no antagonists for these substances has been submitted to clinical testing in Parkinson's disease.

## ►CONCLUSION

During the early stages of Parkinson's disease, response to levodopa is good and patients hardly notice their disease. New symptoms that do not respond well to levodopa make their appearance with time, and people are constantly reminded of their increasing physical handicap. The initial optimism they had experienced when they first started treatment gives way to bitter disappointment and fear for the future. One of the major tasks for scientists and drug researchers is to find treatments that will minimize these late-stage complications. The best way to discover beneficial treatments is to understand their cause. In this respect we have come a long way in our knowledge of the mechanisms that may be involved in late-stage complications. Based on these new findings, the search for new drugs is also progressing at a fairly brisk pace. We must all hope that motor fluctuations will soon be conquered, allowing patients to live better with Parkinson's disease.

# 11

# What Causes Parkinson's Disease?

The cause of premature nerve cell death in Parkinson's disease is still unknown. One of the most intriguing features associated with the group of diseases to which Parkinson's disease belongs, the *neurodegenerative disorders*, is that only certain subsets of nerve cells die in each. It therefore seems likely that the cause of nerve cell death must in each case be linked to something that is unique about the lost cells themselves. Identifying this unique trait could provide important clues to the cause of the disease and is the subject of much research. Since Parkinson's disease usually appears only after the age of 40, theories about the possible causes of Parkinson's disease are often linked to attributes that appear to be unique to substantia nigra nerve cells and to the aging process.

## ►IS PARKINSON'S DISEASE HEREDITARY?

It is important to determine whether Parkinson's disease has a hereditary component—whether it runs in families. If it does, the cause is most probably an abnormal genetic element or gene.

There is evidence both for and against Parkinson's disease being hereditary. Early studies were criticized because the criteria used to decide whether a family member had Parkinson's disease were considered "loose." For example, if a person reports that his now deceased grandfather had a tremor, it is not always easy to know whether it was a symptom of Parkinson's disease or simply a sign of old age. Many studies that try to examine family backgrounds are faced with this dilemma.

Good medical records have shown that Parkinson's disease is hereditary in some families. A few years ago an American neurologist noticed that some of his patients were related and could trace the disease to immigrants from southern Italy. Italian neurologists found members of the same family who also suffered from an inherited form of Parkinson's disease, and still others who emigrated to South America had the disease. This shows that in some instances heredity is more important than environment since people develop the disease wherever they live. Families of this type are unusual but strongly support the possibility that an abnormal gene could cause the disease, at least in some cases.

Evidence *against* a genetic component came from studies of identical twins in which at least one had Parkinson's disease; both twins are affected only about 15 percent of the time, suggesting that factors other than heredity may also be important. However, recent research on inbred animals (which are similar to identical twins) shows that the number of cells in a given organ at birth can vary five-fold from one animal to another; similar differences might exist for the substantia nigra, giving one twin a major advantage over the other.

Faced with this contradictory information, what may be hereditary is the *susceptibility* to an agent such as a virus or toxic substance. Others propose that Parkinson's disease might be due to a genetic defect that can be either inherited or caused by a virus or toxin.

## ►AGING AND PARKINSON'S DISEASE

Because Parkinson's disease usually develops after the age of 40, it might conceivably be the result of an acceleration of the aging process. A mild and progressive loss of nerve cells typically occurs throughout the brain as we age. This is particularly true for substantia nigra nerve cells, whose number decreases steadily with age in everyone. What leads to this slow, normal, age-associated loss of substantia nigra cells is unknown. It might be speculated that we would all develop Parkinson's disease if we lived long enough.

Nerve cell loss in the substantia nigra seems to be accelerated in people with Parkinson's disease. That is, the *process* by which cells are lost might be the same as that causing normal loss, and the abnormality resides in the rapidity with which the process occurs (Figure 11.1).

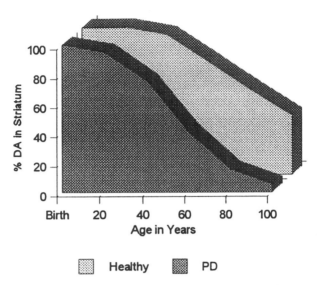

*Figure 11.1.* Schematic representation of the hypothesis that Parkinson's disease (PD) is due to faster than normal aging.

However, the pattern of age-associated cell loss in the substantia nigra of normal individuals differs from that seen in people with Parkinson's disease. For this reason, the cause of nerve cell loss in the disease may differ from the cause of normal age-associated nerve cell loss.

A subject of current debate is whether nerve cell loss in Parkinson's disease occurs slowly over several years or rapidly during a brief period, possibly long before symptoms develop. For example, it has been proposed that some people may suddenly lose large numbers of substantia nigra neurons as the result of exposure to a toxic substance or a virus. Following such an acute loss, perhaps in childhood or young adulthood, these individuals would continue to lose substantia nigra neurons at a normal rate. However, they would reach the critical level for the development of Parkinson's disease— about 70 percent dopamine depletion in the striatum—much earlier than most people as a result of the previous insult. For these people, slowing the normal, age-associated loss of nerve cells would delay the onset of Parkinson's disease.

It has also been suggested that people with Parkinson's disease may simply be born with fewer substantia nerve cells than normal. For such people, too, delaying aging would delay disease onset.

## ►COULD A TOXIN CAUSE PARKINSON'S DISEASE?

As discussed in Chapter 6, the discovery of MPTP led to the development of the monkey model of Parkinson's disease. It also demonstrated that, at least in some instances, parkinsonian symptoms could be the result of a toxin that selectively destroyed substantia nigra nerve cells.

Since that time, researchers have actively looked for substances that could cause substantia nigra neurons to "burn out." One of the first questions that was asked when the search for a toxin started was: When did Parkinson's disease first occur? For example, if the first cases had coincided with the Industrial Revolution, the possibility that the disease is caused by an industrial pollutant would have seemed high. However, a disease identical or similar to Parkinson's disease has clearly existed for thousands of years. If the disease is both ancient *and* due to a toxin, the substance must have been present in the environment for millennia.

Could such a toxin be present in food? Substances found in foods such as cheese, wine, and cocoa (called tetrahydroisoquinolines and betacarbolines) cause nerve cell damage resembling that seen in Parkinson's disease. However, it is unlikely that either substance could be involved in Parkinson's disease because their concentration in foods is very low, and it would seem impossible to ingest toxic quantities of either of these substances. The possibility still exists that some foods contain other, as yet unidentified, compounds that are toxic for substantia nigra neurons. Most scientists feel that this is pure speculation and probably not an area in which to concentrate on discovering the cause of Parkinson's disease.

Other types of toxins considered a possible cause of Parkinson's disease are pesticides and herbicides, some of which have a chemical structure similar to that of MPTP. Farmers using certain types of pesticides, or those drinking well water contaminated by pesticides, might be at risk for developing the disease, and such a linkage has been confirmed in some instances. The brains of some deceased patients showed high levels of pesticide residues.

Another possible source of toxic compounds is an abnormal metabolism that would transform nontoxic substances into toxic ones. A group of liver enzymes, the *cytochrome P450 system*, transforms (metabolizes) substances that we ingest, including medications. There is some evidence that the cytochrome P450 system is different in people with Parkinson's disease compared to the general population, such that a substance that is not toxic for most people could be transformed into a highly toxic substance as a result of abnormal metabolism. In this case, preventing further progression of Parkinson's disease could simply require that patients avoid certain foods, drugs, or environments.

These findings have been questioned because not all subjects who have the P450 abnormality develop Parkinson's disease. As a consequence, a "double hit" theory has been proposed, according to which two defects would be involved in the genesis of Parkinson's disease. Only those who receive both insults (perhaps genetic and environmental) would develop the disease. Having just one defect would not be sufficient.

## ►COULD VIRUSES CAUSE PARKINSON'S DISEASE?

An early hypothesis that Parkinson's disease could be due to a virus was based on cases of progressive parkinsonism that followed *encephalitis*, a brain inflammation caused by a virus. The first observations were of von Economo's encephalitis, which occurred between 1916 and 1926. The virus was never identified, but many suspected it was an influenza virus. Recent results in mice have shown that certain strains of influenza virus selectively colonize substantia nigra nerve cells, favoring the theory that particular types of flu could cause Parkinson's disease.

The recently published case of a patient who suffered from a viral disease complicated by parkinsonism lends additional support to the concept that viruses might cause Parkinson's disease. This patient had an acute and severe viral disease, at the height of which she developed parkinsonian symptoms. MRI scanning showed considerable swelling of the substantia nigra. The patient recovered and the parkinsonian symptoms disappeared. A PET scan after her recovery showed significantly fewer nerve cells in her substantia nigra than in the substantia nigra of other individuals of the same age, suggesting that substantia nigra nerve cells had been destroyed during the acute infectious illness.

Although the patient recovered without any signs of Parkinson's disease, as the years go by she will continue to have normal, age-associated loss of dopamine nerve cells and might eventually develop Parkinson's disease. Some milder viral illnesses might involve minor neuronal loss in the substantia nigra, and several such episodes could result in significant damage to substantia nigra nerve cells, leading to the development of Parkinson's disease.

Everyone has attacks of flu and other viral diseases. The immune system might be weaker in some people, or the barriers that protect the brain might be "leaky," allowing the virus to colonize and destroy substantia nigra nerve cells. It is also possible that viruses affect us differently at different times of our lives. In most people the initial brain lesion caused by the virus probably goes totally unnoticed, but they would reach the critical threshold at which Parkinson's disease becomes apparent when they lose more dopamine nerve cells with age.

## ►CONCLUSION

It is unclear whether Parkinson's disease is hereditary. Although there have been reports of isolated cases of Parkinson's disease caused by a toxic compound (MPTP) or by a virus, there is no proof that the majority of cases are due to a toxin or a virus. Researchers generally agree that Parkinson's disease is most probably the result of both hereditary and environmental factors.

# 12

# Genes and Hormones of Nerve Cell Death

Many scientists hope that identifying the cause of Parkinson's disease will lead to a cure, but this may not be possible if, for example, the cause is a missing protein on the surface of substantia nigra nerve cells. Even if a cure is not possible, another option may be finding ways to stop disease progression based on an understanding of how nerve cells die.

Like all cells, nerve cells can die in one of two ways: they can swell and explode (necrosis) or they can shrink and disappear (apoptosis). In Parkinson's disease, nerve cells appear to die by apoptosis, and blocking this process should stop the disease.

## ► IS IT SAFE TO BLOCK APOPTOSIS?

Apoptosis, also referred to as cell suicide, involves the self-destruction of cells that are no longer needed or are damaged, as is the case in viral infection or cancer. It is under the control of a genetic program that is permanently turned on. To survive, cells require the constant repression of this suicide program by signals from other cells. In other words, cells will die unless they are continually told to live. The life and death of cells thus involves a delicate balance between an internal genetic program telling them to die and external signals telling them to survive.

Apoptosis involves a long cascade of events, and up to a certain stage the process is reversible. Cells that initiate the apoptosis cascade can essentially "change their minds" and live. This can only occur at certain "checkpoints" along the apoptotic cascade. These points are prime targets for drugs to influence apoptosis. The final event on the apoptotic cascade nearly always is a burst of toxic free radicals, extremely toxic substances that kill the cells. Free radicals can also initiate apoptosis; when their levels in a cell become too high, the cell "feels" damaged and self-destructs.

Mature nerve cells do not multiply and lost nerve cells are never replaced. Apoptosis is therefore deleterious to the brain. For other organs of our body, apoptosis is most often a useful phenomenon; it allows for the elimination of cells that have been produced in excess, that have developed improperly, that have sustained genetic damage, or that are infected by viruses. This process is extensively used by the immune system to kill bacteria and viruses as well as abnormal and foreign cells.

The loss of nerve cells by apoptosis occurs in a number of neurodegenerative disorders, including Parkinson's disease. It would therefore seem reasonable to stop their progression by blocking the process. However, a generalized blockade of cell suicide may not be safe because apoptosis is needed to fight infections and cancer. It may be preferable to find drugs that selectively block the process in affected cells. Recent results suggest that this may be possible, but more research is needed to clarify the stimuli that turn apoptosis off only in certain nerve cells, but not in all cells. The following summarizes what is known about the factors that regulate cell suicide.

## ▶ GENETIC CONTROL OF APOPTOSIS

Apoptosis is under genetic control. The genes that control it were first studied in the worm *C. elegans*, in which apoptosis is regulated by a set of at least three genes, two of which *(ced-3* and *ced-4)* cause cell death and a third *(ced-9)* that encodes for a protein that blocks apoptosis.

In humans apoptosis is regulated by a number of genes that are similar to those in the worm, some of which promote apoptosis while others prevent it. One that blocks apoptosis is the *bcl-2* gene, which is similar to *ced-9*. In nerve cells, *bcl-2* decreases the amount of free radicals and thus prevents apoptosis resulting from a variety of factors. Since the concentrations of free radicals in the substantia nigra of people with Parkinson's disease is abnormally high (see Chapter 13), some researchers are searching for ways to inject *bcl-2* genes directly into substantia nigra neurons to help them survive.

The genes that control cell suicide in human cells are now being identified. At least three genes are involved. One of them, *p53*, codes for a protein that prevents the formation of the *bcl-2* protein, possibly by switching off the *bcl-2* gene. The gene plays a major role in deciding whether a cell should commit apoptosis. It receives signals from various parts of the cell that reflect its health, and it orders apoptosis if it detects anything threatening, such as cancer or infection. Until recently cancer was thought to be due to excessive cell proliferation, but recent research has shown that many human cancers involve an inability to commit apoptosis due to alterations in the *p53* gene. Perhaps other not yet identified alterations in the *p53* gene lead cells to commit apoptosis too easily.

Another "killer" gene is one that codes for an enzyme called ICE (interleukin-1-β converting enzyme). Interleukin-1-β, a protein made by many cells of the body, is a powerful promoter of apoptosis. Because it is such a dangerous compound, cells do not directly produce interleukin-1-β; rather they make an inactive precursor that is converted to interleukin-1-β by ICE.

A third suicide gene codes for the enzyme *CPP-32*, which disables the mechanisms involved in gene surveillance and repair. Cells that can no longer repair their genes are prone to suicide, and *CPP-32* may be more relevant to apoptosis than ICE. Drugs that block the activity of *CPP-32* might stop apoptosis in a number of diseases.

Many other genes are probably involved in the regulation of apoptosis, and rapid progress is being made in understanding the mystery of cell suicide.

## ►VIRUSES AND APOPTOSIS

Certain viruses may be able to teach us how to prevent apoptosis. Cells that become infected by a virus normally commit suicide, thus killing the virus and preventing other cells from becoming infected. *Baculovirus*, which infects insects, contains a gene called *p35*, which prevents the cell from committing suicide. The infected cell survives and viral production is enhanced 200- to 15,000-fold. The mechanism by which *p35* prevents apoptosis is not yet fully understood, but it is known to be different from that of *bcl-2* and may involve inhibition of the enzyme ICE. Some researchers have suggested inserting *p35* genes into the substantia nigra to stop the progression of Parkinson's disease.

## ►SURVIVAL SIGNALS: NEUROTROPHIC FACTORS

Nerve cells have an ovoid shape in early stages of development. As they mature, each extends a single long process known as an axon until it makes contact with its target. The human brain has a complex system of connections between nerve cells. Many developing neurons are faced with the daunting task of sending their axons to distant targets through an intricate obstacle course of other cells and growing axons. If a nerve cell sends its axons to the wrong target, it dies by apoptosis, ensuring that connections between nerve cells in the mature brain are nearly always correct.

When researchers removed a target tissue before axons reached it (Figure 12.1), axons arrived in the target region but then stopped growing and died. The only explanation was that the target tissue liberated a factor that promoted survival and growth of the incoming nerve cell. This factor had to be specific for both the target tissue and the nerve cell. It was termed a *neurotrophic* factor because it caused nerve cells to survive, grow, and mature. The first such factor to be identified was nerve growth factor (NGF), which acts on many different kinds of nerve cells. Many others have since been discovered.

Neurotrophic factors were first thought of as substances whose only function was to drive and organize early brain development, but they are equally involved in the survival of adult neurons. For example, in adult animals certain sets of nerve cells begin to undergo apoptosis when their neurotrophic factors are inactivated or removed. When it was found that nerve cells die by apoptosis in Parkinson's disease, many speculated that the disease might be due to a loss of one or more neurotrophic factors. If so, replacement of the missing factor(s) could probably block disease progression. Interest in these factors reached a high point when it was found that GDNF (glial-cell-line-derived-neurotrophic factor) prevents adult substantia nigra nerve cells from undergoing apoptosis.

Neurotrophic factors exert their effects by interacting with receptors on the outer surface of nerve cells that have an outer unit, which recognizes and binds their neurotrophic factor, as well as an inner unit (Figure 12.2). When the outer unit is occupied by its neurotrophic factor, the inner unit changes so as to initiate a chain reaction of signals and events that result in nerve cell growth, maturation, and survival. Following interaction with their receptor, neurotrophic factors are taken up into the axon and transported to the nerve cell body, often over a considerable distance. It is not yet known what they do when they travel up the axon or what their role is after they reach the nerve cell body.

Adult nerve cells are usually under the influence of several neurotrophic factors, including those secreted by their target tissues, those secreted by neighboring cells, and those produced by glial cells. Adult neurons also make neurotrophic factors that are liberated into the synaptic cleft, where they

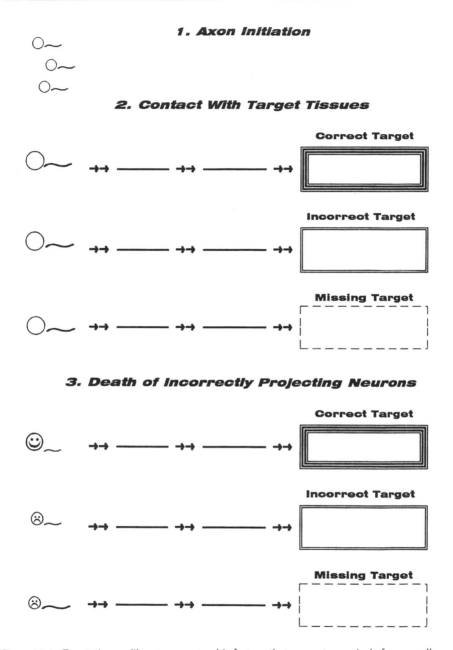

*Figure 12.1.* Target tissues liberate neurotrophic factors that promote survival of nerve cells.

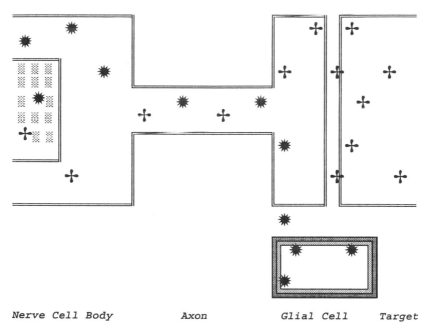

Nerve Cell Body              Axon              Glial Cell      Target

*Figure 12.2.* Schematic representation of the liberation of neurotrophic factors by target tissue (✛) or by glial cells (✳).Once liberated, these factors cross the synapse and interact with specific receptors.

stimulate their own neurotrophic receptors. Factors liberated by blood cells and other types of cells also promote nerve cell survival.

## ►NEUROTROPHIC FACTORS AND PARKINSON'S DISEASE

Different types of nerve cells respond to different neurotrophic factors. Two of these play an important role in the development and survival of substantia nigra neurons. BDNF (brain-derived neurotrophic factor) acts mainly during early development. It is liberated by substantia nigra nerve cells and is thus an example of a neurotrophic factor that is liberated by and acts on neighboring nerve cells. GDNF is liberated by glial cells and may play a major role in the survival of adult substantia nigra neurons.

As is true for all nerve cells, adult substantia nigra neurons die when their axons are "cut," perhaps because they no longer receive survival messages from their target tissues. In adult rats most substantia nigra neurons can be protected from death by treatment with GDNF at the same time as their axons are cut, proving that GDNF can protect nerve cells from apoptosis.

The protective effect of GDNF was also studied in a situation more similar to Parkinson's disease, in which mouse substantia nigra cells were destroyed by MPTP. One group of mice was treated with GDNF while nerve cells were simultaneously treated with MPTP, whereas a second group received only MPTP. The number of substantia nigra nerve cells destroyed was considerably lower in the group that received GDNF. When its "rescue" effects were studied by treating mice with GDNF several days after their nerve cells had been injured, GDNF still protected a substantial number of substantia nigra neurons, indicating that it can rescue nerve cells even after they have turned on their suicide program.

Rats treated with GDNF four weeks after their substantia nigra nerve cells were destroyed with 6-hydroxydopamine developed normal dopamine neurons in their lesioned substantia nigra. The finding suggests that GDNF might cause nerve cells to regrow after they have been destroyed. However, it is also possible that nerve cells were not quite dead four weeks after 6-hydroxydopamine was administered and that GDNF was able to rescue them.

When GDNF was administered to monkeys three months after substantia nigra nerve cells were destroyed by MPTP, at a time when the lesion was complete and fixed, there was some improvement in bradykinesia, rigidity, and postural instability, as well as a slight increase in dopamine levels in the striatum. The results did not qualify as spectacular, perhaps because by the time GDNF was administered virtually all nerve cells had died. Most agree that GDNF is more likely to rescue dying nerve cells rather than to cause new nerve cells to grow.

## ▶ GDNF FOR THE TREATMENT OF PARKINSON'S DISEASE

Much work is needed before GDNF or any other neurotrophic factor can be used routinely in humans. One major problem that must be overcome is the route of administration. Neurotrophic factors cannot be given orally because they are destroyed in the stomach; nor can they be injected intravenously because they are not taken up in the brain. Neurotrophic factors are administered directly into the brain in animals, which may not be practical or even possible in humans. A clinical trial in which GDNF is injected into the brain once a month has started in patients with Parkinson's disease.

One way to deliver GDNF directly to the substantia nigra neurons would be to implant genetically engineered cells that produce the desired neurotrophic factor into the substantia nigra (see Chapter 14). This type of approach has the advantage of delivering GDNF only to "sick" neurons. Another approach would be to find drugs that increase the production of

GDNF by glial cells. Antidepressants have been shown to increase the production of BDNF, another growth factor for substantia nigra nerve cells, but no drug has yet been shown to increase GDNF production

A better alternative may be to find substances that stimulate GDNF receptors. Such compounds might be small molecules that are absorbed from the bowel and taken up by the brain, making it possible to treat patients orally. The recent discovery of the GDNF receptor is a major advance for this type of approach.

Numerous other issues must be considered. The possibility exists that Parkinson's disease is due to a lack of response to neurotrophic factors rather than to their absence. Another issue is the risk of neuronal overgrowth, which might be dose-dependent. Identifying the correct dose of neurotrophic factor will not be easy. Finally, it will be crucial to show that the effects are permanent. Other neurotrophic factors have been reported to rescue nerve cells, but their effects last only a short time.

In conclusion, the discovery that neurotrophic factors are essential for the survival of adult nerve cells provides new clues in the search for treatments to halt the progression of Parkinson's disease, but a great deal more research is needed before these discoveries can lead to new therapies

## ▶ DEATH SIGNALS: PROINFLAMMATORY CYTOKINES PROMOTE APOPTOSIS

In addition to being controlled by a genetic program and survival signals, apoptosis is also influenced by many other chemical messengers, several of which might be involved in Parkinson's disease. A group of substances called *proinflammatory cytokines* might be of particular relevance in a number of neurodegenerative disorders, including Parkinson's disease, especially if the disease is caused by a virus.

Cytokines are messenger molecules produced by those cells throughout the body that form the immune system and work together to defend against invasion by foreign substances. The immune system seeks and destroys infectious agents such as bacteria, viruses, parasites, or fungi; it destroys the body's own cells when they become abnormal, as is the case with cancer cells; and it destroys normal cells that come from another person, as with transplanted organs or tissues.

The immune system has the remarkable ability to distinguish between the body's own cells and proteins, termed *self*, and foreign cells and proteins, termed *non-self*. The immune system swings into action as soon as it recognizes a foreign cell or protein and destroys the intruder. The immune system is extremely complex; it can recognize millions of different enemies and it can produce cells, antibodies, and secretions that match each one and destroy it. The cells of the immune system communicate with each other either by direct contact or by releasing chemical messengers, called *cytokines*. Immune cells called *microglia* are also present in the brain.

The messages carried by cytokines usually deal with cell growth, differentiation, survival, or death. Most cytokines are secreted outside the cells that make them and act on neighboring cells. Given their potency, it is not surprising that the production and action of cytokines are tightly and elaborately controlled. With respect to the control of cell survival and death, it is believed that there is a network of positive (anti-suicide) and negative (pro-suicide) cytokines and that this network is controlled by a complex system of inhibitors and inducers. The combined action of these substances leads to an overall effect that causes cells to live or die. An imbalance in the cytokine network has the potential to induce disease.

## ►CYTOKINE FAMILIES

Many cytokines have been identified during the past few years, and they have been grouped into several large families, including an important group know as the interleukins. One of them, interleukin-1-β, is thought to be involved in Alzheimer's disease. Interleukin-1-β is primarily a pro-suicide cytokine. Cells that produce it make an inactive precursor that is converted to active interleukin-1-β by the enzyme ICE. The current view is that many cells contain the inactive precursor of interleukin-1-β and that stimulation of the gene that codes for ICE leads to the formation of active interleukin-1-β, and consequently to apoptosis. A characteristic of cytokine families is that its members may have opposing effects; for example, other interleukins block the effects of interleukin-1-β. Abnormal cell death may occur if the balance between these cytokines is disrupted.

A second family of cytokines is the interferons. There are at least three different types of interferons (interferon-α, interferon-β, and interferon-γ). As with interleukins, there is a subtle equilibrium between their effects. Interferon-γ is secreted by the cells of the immune system in response to germs, especially viruses, and interferon-β counterbalances this effect. Multiple sclerosis may be caused by an excessive production of interferon-γ in response to viral diseases (as if the cells of the immune system overreact), and treatment with interferon-β may be beneficial.

Tumor-necrosing-factor-α (TNF-α) belongs to a third family of cytokines. Viruses can cause many different types of cells to produce and secrete this powerful promoter of cell suicide. In the brain, however, it may have the opposite effect and may prevent nerve cells from committing apoptosis. Its levels are abnormally high in the substantia nigra of patients with Parkinson's disease, but it is unclear whether this causes nerve cells to commit suicide or whether it represents an attempt by the brain to rescue dying nerve cells by having the opposite effect of preventing nerve cells from committing apoptosis.

### Cytokine Receptors

Cytokines exert their effects by interacting with receptors located on the cell surface that function very much like receptors for neurotrophic factors. They contain two functional units, one on the outer surface of the cell, to which the cytokine binds, and one inside the cell. A cytokine that binds to the outer unit of its receptor changes the inner unit, which in turn triggers a cascade of signals and events inside the cell that causes either cell death or cell growth and survival.

### Cytokine Antagonists

Several naturally occurring substances block the effect of cytokines, giving us clues in the search of drugs that block the effects of pro-apoptosis cytokines. For example, certain brain cells make a substance that binds to the outer unit of the interleukin-1-β receptor without changing the inner unit, and therefore without causing any of the effects of interleukin-1-β. This receptor antagonist prevents interleukin-1-β from binding to its receptor, and thus protects nerve cells from the effects of the cytokine. Little is known about this substance, but decreased amounts of interleukin-1-β antagonist might contribute to the appearance of certain neurodegenerative diseases.

Another example of cytokine antagonists are proteins that are made and secreted into the blood stream by a number of cells and bind to cytokines. Although some of these binding proteins may be carriers of cytokines, extending their duration and radius of action, others may neutralize cytokines and protect cells against excessive amounts.

Infectious agents, especially certain viruses, can subvert the cytokine network to their own ends and thus provide clues about how to block cytokines. Viruses typically penetrate a cell and cause it to make substances that it does not usually produce. Many viruses cause cells to produce cytokine inhibitors. For example, vaccinia and cowpox viruses induce cells to make and secrete a protein that neutralizes interleukin-1-β, while others cause cells to produce and release proteins that neutralize TNF-α. Since both these cytokines are powerful germ killers, these inhibitors probably protect viruses against the immune system.

## TREATMENTS TO BLOCK CYTOKINES

The search for drugs that affect the cytokine network has just begun, but initial results are encouraging. As always, when a possible cause for a disease is identified, scientists start by looking to see if there is any commercially available drug that might block it.

Glucocorticoids, such as those used to treat rheumatoid arthritis, are potent inhibitors of many cytokines, notably interleukin-1-β. Other anti-inflammatory drugs, such as aspirin, also prevent many of the effects of cytokines. One study showed a greatly reduced risk of Alzheimer's disease in people treated with anti-inflammatory drugs (usually for arthritis), perhaps because increased levels of interleukin-1-β are the cause of nerve cell loss in Alzheimer's disease. A number of available drugs block the production of TNF-α, but it is unclear whether this is desirable since this cytokine may have anti-suicide effects in the brain. Finally, certain dietary modifications influence cytokine production and actions. For example, supplementation with omega-3-fatty acids inhibits many of the effects of interleukin-1-β in rats.

In addition to studying known drugs, scientists are actively looking for new ones that would block some of the effects of killer cytokines or enhance the effects of those that promote cell survival. Of key importance will be the development of agents that act locally within the brain regions affected by Parkinson's disease since a generalized inhibition of pro-suicide cytokines could increase the risk of infections and other problems.

## CONCLUSION

Cell survival is the result of many opposing forces. Cells are under the control of a genetic program that continually tells them to self-destruct, but they also receive signals that tell them to live. Cell survival is the result of a delicate balance between these signals. Any abnormality in this complex signaling system can lead to disease. If cells stop paying attention to death messages, the risk may be cancer. If they do not listen to or do not receive survival messages, the risk may be arthritis or neurodegenerative disorders.

Nerve cells deprived of their specific neurotrophic factors turn on their apoptosis program and die within a few hours. A number of neurodegenerative disorders, including Parkinson's disease, could be due to the absence of a specific neurotrophic factor. Giving patients the missing factor or drugs that mimic its effects might rescue nerve cells and stop the progression of the neurodegenerative disease.

Neurotrophic factors may also be useful if nerve cell death is due to excessive death signals rather than to a loss of survival signals. One way to protect the cell would be to reduce these signals. Another would be to increase the level of survival signals by administering neurotrophic factors or drugs that mimic their effects. Treatment with neurotrophic factors may be the proper approach whether cell death is due to insufficient amounts of survival signals or to excessive amounts of death signals. Another advantage of neurotrophic factors is their selectivity; since each promotes the survival of only certain cell types, the risk associated with generalized inhibition of cell suicide can be avoided.

As the mechanisms that lead to apoptosis become understood, the number of targets for anti-apoptosis drugs will increase and with it the hope to be able one day to stop disabling diseases such as Parkinson's disease.

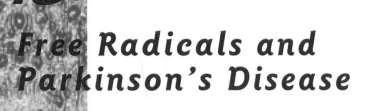

# 13

# Free Radicals and Parkinson's Disease

In Chapter 12 we showed that in each cell apoptosis is under the control of an internal genetic program and external signals, which trigger cascades of events that take place inside the cell and ultimately lead to its death. Little is yet known about these apoptotic cascades except that they involve a complex chain of events and that different triggers involve slightly different cascades. The last event of the apoptotic cascade most often is an explosion of free radicals that kills the cell. Free radicals can also *initiate* apoptosis by mechanisms that are not entirely clear, but cells that contain high levels of free radicals self-destruct as if they "felt" damaged. Certain substances, such as iron, increase the toxicity of free radicals and promote apoptosis.

Several lines of evidence suggest that increased concentrations of free radicals in the substantia nigra may be the cause of nerve cell death in Parkinson's disease. As a consequence, drugs that remove free radicals from nerve cells might help slow disease progression.

Free radicals are extremely toxic substances that are formed continuously by all cells of the human body as a consequence of normal functioning, especially by processes such as respiration, tissue repair, and fighting infections. For example, a group of enzymes called *oxidases* continuously generate free radicals. Mitochondria, the "lungs" of all cells, are another major source; they "breathe in" oxygen and "breathe out" free radicals and produce energy for the cells in the process. Mitochondria are therefore not only the "lungs" of the cells, but also little energy factories that produce toxic byproducts.

Free radicals are normally "scavenged" by a complex system of enzymes that protect the cells of the body, often called *antioxidant enzymes*. A number of antioxidant compounds that include vitamins C and E also scavenge free radicals. Free radicals that are not immediately scavenged travel a short distance within the cell, damaging it in the process. The action of antioxidants on free radicals is comparable to that of a sponge on water—antioxidants "mop up" free radicals and neutralize them as soon as they are formed. Scavenging systems are the same in all the cells of the body, but the levels of scavenging enzymes and antioxidants are higher in some cells than in others. An excess of free radicals can be due to a defective scavenging system, an overproduction of free radicals, or a combination of both.

## ►NEURONS ARE VERY SENSITIVE TO FREE RADICALS

Since free radicals are produced in all cells all the time, one would expect a "free radical disease" to affect all cells of the body, but some cells are more vulnerable to free radicals than others. Neurons are especially sensitive to free radicals because the levels of scavenging enzymes in the brain are low. Moreover, unlike other cells, nerve cells obtain nearly all their energy from mitochondria. Mitochondria are thus very active in nerve cells and produce a large number of free radicals. The shape and chemical composition of nerve cells also make them especially sensitive to free radical damage. Neurons have long, thin extensions (axons and dendrites) and small cell bodies. Their high ratio of "skin" (outer membrane) to volume is much greater than that of other cell types, increasing the risk of free radical damage (Figure 13.1).

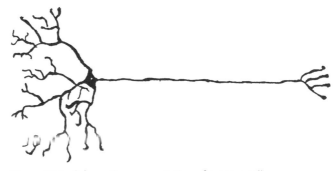

*Figure 13.1.* Schematic representation of a nerve cell.

Additionally, the brain has a high content of lipids, especially polyunsaturated fatty acids, which are prime targets for free radical damage.

This explains why neurons are more vulnerable to free radicals than many other cells in the body, but does not explain why free radicals would cause only certain neurons to burn out in a condition such as Parkinson's disease. Differences between neurons could explain selective vulnerabilities. For example, substantia nigra neurons appear to contain more free radicals than other neurons because the degradation of levodopa and dopamine liberates them, which might be related to the development of Parkinson's disease (Figure 13.2).

Substantia nigra neurons slowly and over a period of some years produce a substance called *neuromelanin* via a process that involves the liberation of free radicals. Unlike other nerve cells that make dopamine, substantia nigra neurons also contain high levels of iron, which increases the toxicity of free radicals.

Thus, Parkinson's disease could be due to either a slight generalized defect in free radical scavenging processes, a modest and generalized overproduction of free radicals, or a slow accumulation of iron. Most cells survive this problem without any difficulty, but substantia nigra neurons already have a lot of free radicals to deal with and cannot cope with any additional increase. Substantia nigra nerve cells therefore slowly burn out, with symptoms of Parkinson's disease developing when dopamine levels in the striatum are decreased by more than 80 percent.

## ▶FREE RADICALS AND FAMILIAL LOU GEHRIG'S DISEASE

In 1994 a breakthrough discovery was made for the familial form of amyotrophic lateral sclerosis (ALS or Lou Gehrig's disease). Scientists looking for the abnormal feature that was genetically transmitted to cause the disease found that one of the enzymes involved in free radical scavenging,

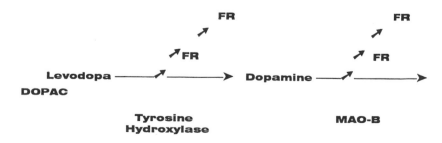

*Figure 13.2.* Free radicals (FR) are formed as a result of the degradation of levodopa and dopamine.

super-oxide-dismutase (SOD), did not scavenge free radicals properly. Family members who had the abnormal enzyme also had the disease. The enzyme defect was due to an abnormal gene that codes for SOD. This discovery shows that at least one form of neurodegenerative disease is probably caused by free radicals and has greatly encouraged the search for new drugs that scavenge them. However, a note of caution must be made: SOD does more than scavenge free radicals; it also traps copper. Lou Gehrig's disease could therefore be due to an excessive amount of copper in certain nerve cells rather than to an overload in free radicals.

## ▶ARE FREE RADICALS INVOLVED IN PARKINSON'S DISEASE?

Detecting free radicals is difficult because of their highly reactive and transient nature. It is almost impossible to obtain direct proof of an overload of free radicals in the substantia nigra of people who have Parkinson's disease. However, increasing indirect evidence suggests that free radicals are at least partly involved in nerve cell damage in this region. One of the first signs of free radical damage to membranes is the formation of a compound called cholesterol-lipid-hydro-peroxide. Its levels are ten times higher than normal in the substantia nigra of people with Parkinson's disease. Markers of free radical damage called lipid peroxides and 8-hydroxy-deoxyguanosine are also abnormally high in the substantia nigra of people with Parkinson's disease.

Another indication that free radicals may play a role in the genesis of Parkinson's disease is that levels of glutathione, a marker of how well free radicals are scavenged, are reduced in the substantia nigra of patients with early Parkinson's disease who have not yet received levodopa. Low levels of glutathione suggest that their substantia nigra cells do not scavenge free radicals normally. Additionally, animal experiments have shown that compounds that increase free radical formation cause lesions of substantia nigra neurons similar to those observed in Parkinson's disease.

## ▶MITOCHONDRIAL ABNORMALITIES INCREASE THE FREE RADICAL LOAD IN PARKINSON'S DISEASE

The discovery of an abnormality in the mitochondria of people with Parkinson's disease is another reason to believe that free radicals are central to its development. Because the abnormality is found *only* in the substantia nigra, many people think it may be the cause of the disease. It consists of a partial loss of a subunit of the mitochondria called *complex-1*, as a result of which the mitochondria do not produce enough energy. Because of energy failure, the cell cannot make as many free radical scavengers as it should, and levels of free radicals rise dangerously. Complex-1 malfunction has also been reported in people with other neurodegenerative disorders, including Huntington's disease and Alzheimer's disease. In Parkinson's disease, complex-1 deficiency is found only in the substantia nigra. It has not yet been determined if the deficit affects nerve cells, glial cells, or both. The abnormality could be either genetically inherited or induced by toxic substances.

Free radicals generated by mitochondria destroy parts of complex-1 if they are not immediately scavenged. Thus, complex-1 abnormalities are not only the cause but also the consequence of free radical damage. A vicious circle is initiated, whereby a deficiency in mitochondrial complex-1 leads to increased free radical levels, which in turn cause more damage to complex-1. Cells that are deficient in complex-1, or in which complex-1 is "paralyzed," ultimately die by apoptosis.

Complex-1 deficiency in the substantia nigra thus could be the primary cause of Parkinson's disease or it might be secondary to free radical overload. Even if this mitochondrial abnormality is only a secondary event, it most likely exacerbates the deleterious effects of free radicals and thereby accelerates the course of Parkinson's disease.

## ▶ MPTP TOXICITY INVOLVES COMPLEX-1

MPTP lesions dopamine cells by a process that involves complex-1 inactivation (Figure 13.3). MPTP is transformed into the highly toxic MPP+ in glial cells. It leaves the glial cell and is taken up specifically by dopamine neurons,

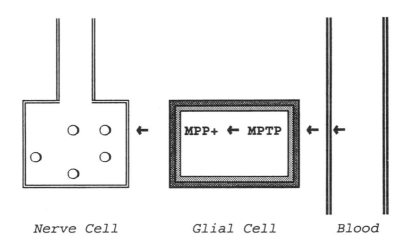

Nerve Cell          Glial Cell          Blood

*Figure 13.3.* Schematic representation of the mechanism by which MPTP destroys neurons. MPP+ is taken up by dopamine uptake site on substantia nigra nerve cell.

where it "paralyzes" complex-1. This selective uptake explains why only dopamine neurons are destroyed. The discovery that MPTP causes nerve cell lesions identical to those of Parkinson's disease by damaging complex-1 in the mitochondria lends further support to the theory that an abnormality of this substance is the cause of Parkinson's disease.

Since excess free radicals might be either the primary cause of or a secondary aggravating factor for Parkinson's disease, antioxidants might slow its progression. However, the antioxidant vitamin E does not slow the progression of Parkinson's disease. This might mean that free radicals are not involved or that scavenging them will not be helpful. It may simply reflect the fact that vitamin E does not penetrate the brain very well.

Because free radicals are formed in localized areas of the cell such as the mitochondria, a scavenger would have to be in the exact spot in the cell where excess free radicals are formed in order to prevent damage; simply entering the brain would not be sufficient. Since the source of excess free radicals in Parkinson's disease has not yet been identified, we do not know where in the nerve cell the free radical scavenger must act.

It has been difficult to find free radical scavengers that enter the brain, and those few that do are usually tested in cases of stroke and head trauma. It is hard to show that a drug is beneficial for these conditions. A small number of free radical scavengers that do enter the brain were discovered (usually by chance), studied in patients with stroke or head trauma, and not found to be effective. They were not followed up for their potential usefulness in other diseases, partly because evidence pointing toward the involvement of free radicals in neurodegenerative disorders is very recent.

To the best of our knowledge, only one free radical scavenger, OPC-14117, is currently being tested in people with Parkinson's disease. Clinical trials with this compound are ongoing in the United States. In laboratory experiments, this drug scavenges free radicals with a potency comparable to that of vitamin E. OPC-14117 also protects neurons from toxins that kill substantia nigra neurons. When given orally to animals, it readily penetrates the brain, where its levels are close to five times higher than in the bloodstream. Several other free radical scavengers are currently being tested in animals, and some may soon become available for clinical testing.

## ▶ IRON ACCUMULATION INCREASES FREE RADICAL TOXICITY IN PARKINSON'S DISEASE

The brain contains substantially more iron than any other metal. Its distribution is uneven, with particularly high levels in the substantia nigra. The exact function of iron in the brain is unknown, but it is thought to be necessary for normal brain function, especially for memory and learning. Iron levels normally increase with age in the substantia nigra, but they are particularly high in people with Parkinson's disease. Iron is known to promote apoptosis, most likely because it increases the toxicity of free radicals, so high concentrations of iron might be related to nerve cell loss in Parkinson's disease.

High iron levels could also be a consequence of nerve cell death, rather than its cause, because iron is liberated when substantia nigra nerve cells die. The increase could make remaining neurons more vulnerable to free radical damage, accelerating the progression of disease.

Drugs called *iron chelators* bind iron and force its elimination in the urine. In animals chelators such as deferoxamine slow the degeneration of substantia nigra neurons caused by the toxic substance 6-hydroxydopamine. Its effects in Parkinson's disease have not been tested, and to the best of our knowledge there is no clinical trial ongoing with this drug to see if it might slow disease progression. One problem may be to find iron chelators that act selectively for the brain, since depleting iron from the entire body would have harmful effects because, for example, iron plays an important role in red blood cells.

## ►GLUTAMATE INCREASES FREE RADICAL LOAD

Another way to reduce oxidative stress is to decrease the formation of free radicals. In the substantia nigra free radicals are generated through many processes. For example, the degradation of dopamine by the enzyme MAO-B (monoamine oxidase type B) liberates free radicals. Many believe that selegiline (Eldepryl®), which blocks MAO-B, may slow the progression of Parkinson's disease because it decreases free radical load in the substantia nigra. Other MAO-B inhibitors are currently being tested in patients, but recent reports of possible long-term toxicity of selegiline has somewhat dampened the enthusiasm of researchers for this type of drug. Another cause of free radical formation in the substantia nigra is the stimulation of glutamate receptors.

### Glutamate Is a Neurotransmitter

Glutamate has many functions in the brain. Like dopamine, glutamate is a neurotransmitter. It is synthesized in nerve terminals, stored in small vesicles, and released as needed in the synaptic cleft (Figure 13.4). It crosses the synaptic cleft and interacts with "receptors" located on the opposite side of the synapse. When glutamate interacts with its receptors, it turns on a cascade of events that leads to its effects and the production of free radicals.

High concentrations of glutamate in the synaptic cleft are toxic for nerve cells. It is therefore imperative that it be removed as soon as it has finished

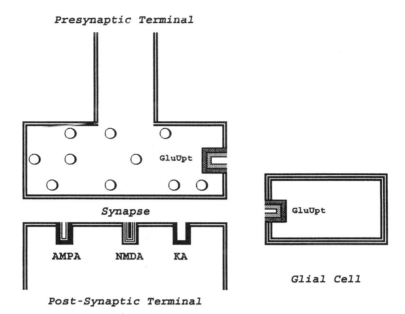

*Figure 13.4.* Schematic diagram of a glutamate synapse. Glutamate is stored in small vesicles (O) and liberated in the synaptic cleft as needed. It crosses the synaptic cleft and interacts with its receptors (nerve cells do not necessarily carry all types of glutamate receptors; they may have only one or two types of receptors). When glutamate has finished interacting with its receptors, it is "pumped" out of the synaptic cleft by a powerful uptake mechanism on glial cells and nerve endings (GluUpt).

interacting with its receptors. Its removal is accomplished by re-uptake in the nerve terminal from which it was liberated and uptake into glial cells that surround the synaptic cleft (Figure 13.4). A defect of this uptake mechanism may be the cause of the nonfamilial form of amyotrophic lateral sclerosis (Lou Gehrig's disease).

The mechanism by which excessive glutamate causes nerve cell death is not completely known. It seems to involve mainly the NMDA receptor, and many lines of evidence point toward its killing nerve cells by causing increased entry of calcium and an overproduction of free radicals. In animals drugs that scavenge free radicals block the toxicity of glutamate, lending further support to the concept that glutamate toxicity is mediated by free radical overload.

### Glutamate and Parkinson's Disease

At present glutamate toxicity is not considered to be the primary cause of Parkinson's disease, but scientists agree that glutamate could cause the disease to progress more rapidly. This belief is based on the following supposition. Let us assume that Parkinson's disease is due to an abnormality in substantia nigra mitochondria, with a partial loss of complex-1. Consequently, substantia nigra nerve cells do not scavenge free radicals well. Usual, everyday-type stimulation of glutamate receptors causes a moderate increase in free radical load. This normally would not be a problem. In the case of a complex-1 deficiency, however, nerve cells cannot protect themselves from surges in free radical levels. From a practical standpoint, it may take many years before scientists find a way to replace missing pieces of complex-1. In the meantime, blocking glutamate receptors in the substantia nigra may protect nerve cells.

A number of observations support this theory. For example, drugs that block the NMDA receptor attenuate the deleterious effects of toxic substances such as MPP+, which causes lesions of complex-1 in the mitochondria similar to those observed in patients with Parkinson's disease. Another result that favors the aggravating role of glutamate in Parkinson's disease is provided by experiments conducted in rats. Nerve cells located in a brain region called the subthalamic nucleus use glutamate as their neurotransmitter. These nerve cells send axons (projections) that liberate glutamate in the substantia nigra. In rats, paralyzing the subthalamic nucleus by high frequency electrical stimulation prevents the liberation of glutamate in the substantia nigra and protects neurons from the toxic effects of 6-hydroxydopamine, a toxin that kills nerve cells by generating free radicals, not by interfering with the glutamate transmission. This protective role of high frequency electrical stimulation is a good example of how blocking glutamate transmission can be beneficial even in situations in which nerve cell death is not primarily due to glutamate.

### Glutamate Receptors

Unlike dopamine, which acts as a neurotransmitter for only a small number of neurons, glutamate is a neurotransmitter for approximately 40 percent of brain nerve cells. It is thought that glutamate plays a major role in many vital processes, such as control of blood pressure, respiration, and alertness, as well as in functions that serve intelligence, such as learning and memory. Glutamate is also a major neurotransmitter in the spinal cord, where it is essential for normal motor function. Given the widespread distribution of glutamate and the critical functions it serves, it is not surprising that drugs that block glutamate have many serious side effects. Research is focusing on the discovery of drugs that act only in specific brain areas to minimize side effects due to generalized inhibition of glutamate transmission. In Parkinson's disease, the goal is to discover drugs that act mainly in the substantia nigra.

The interaction of glutamate with its receptors causes either a channel for sodium or a channel for calcium to open (Figure 13.5). Entry of sodium, calcium, or both into the nerve cell is the first step in a complicated cascade of events that leads to the effects of glutamate, which if excessive lead to toxicity. Glutamate transmission can be blocked in several ways. One of glutamate's many receptors can be blocked, or the channels controlled by glutamate receptors can be "plugged."

Nearly every nerve cell in the brain carries glutamate receptors, but its effects vary tremendously from one nerve cell to another because there are many different glutamate receptors. Glutamate receptors are made of several subunits, and receptor diversity is further increased by the many ways in which they can associate. Some subunits are found nearly exclusively in certain brain regions, and targeting them would lead to drugs that act mainly in one specific brain region.

### NMDA Receptors

Unlike the other glutamate receptors, the NMDA receptor controls a channel that is highly permeable to calcium. It is therefore thought to be the receptor most involved in the neurotoxicity of glutamate, and drugs to prevent nerve cell death are usually directed at this receptor, which is quite complex and offers several targets for drugs (Figure 13.6).

In addition to a binding site for glutamate (the NMDA site), there is also a binding site for glycine. Both sites must be occupied for the associated channel to open, and blocking either prevents channel opening. Additionally, the receptor contains a modulatory site that binds polyamines. Blocking this site does not prevent channel opening but makes it more difficult. Many believe that this is the best site to target for neuroprotective drugs because its

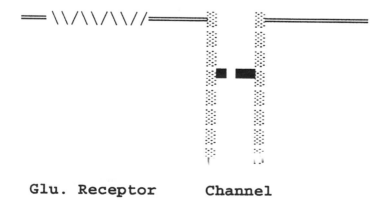

**Glu. Receptor          Channel**

*Figure 13.5.* Glutamate receptors control the opening of sodium or calcium channels

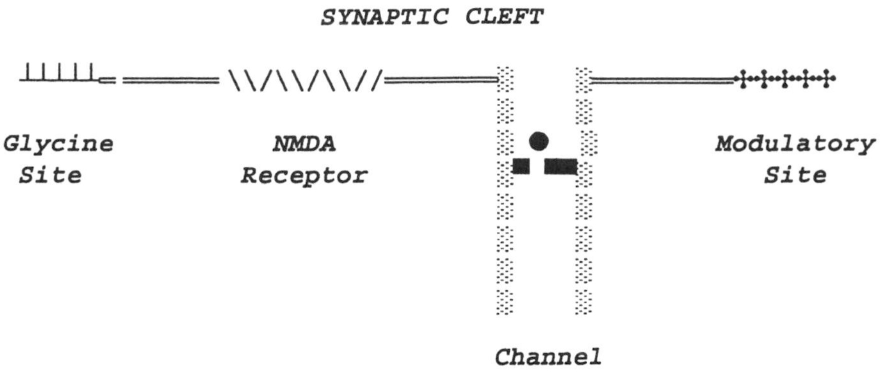

SYNAPTIC CLEFT

Glycine
Site

NMDA
Receptor

Modulatory
Site

Channel

Figure 13.6. Schematic representation of an NMDA receptor. At rest, the NMDA channel is blocked by magnesium.

inhibition does not completely block NMDA function, which is critical for many processes, notably memory.

One of the most unique features of the NMDA receptor is that at rest its associated channel is blocked by magnesium, which acts like a plug preventing calcium from flowing through the channel. When glutamate is liberated into the synaptic cleft, it binds to the AMPA and the NMDA receptors. Binding to the NMDA receptor is useless because the NMDA channel is plugged by magnesium. Binding to the AMPA causes the magnesium plug to pop out. The NMDA receptor then becomes operational, calcium flows into the nerve cell, and free radicals are generated.

### NMDA Receptor Antagonists

When the role of the NMDA receptor in glutamate toxicity was recognized, researchers began looking for drugs that could block its receptor. They tested thousands of old drugs in experiments conducted in test tubes and discovered almost by chance that a drug called *dextromethorphan* blocks the NMDA receptor. This drug became available more than 30 years ago as an anti-cough medication and is still extensively used for this indication. Following the discovery that dextromethorphan is an NMDA antagonist, researchers tested it in people with neurodegenerative disorders to see if they could slow or stop disease progression. The doses of dextromethorphan that are used to prevent coughing are much lower than the doses that are needed to block NMDA receptors in the brain. Researchers therefore tried to use higher doses of dextromethorphan, but patients complained of sedation (sleepiness) at doses that were still lower than those thought to be required to fully block NMDA receptors. In general, many of the currently available NMDA antagonists induce side effects, such as sedation, hypotension, and mental changes, that preclude their use in patients with Parkinson's disease. These side effects are most probably due to widespread inhibition of NMDA receptors.

Amantadine (Symmetrel®)is another older drug that has recently been reported to slow the progression of Parkinson's disease and has therefore attracted renewed interest. It originally became available in Europe as an effective antiviral agent against A2 Asian influenza. In 1969 it was found to improve the symptoms of Parkinson's disease in a patient who had flu. Several clinical trials confirmed this initial observation and by the late 1970s amantadine was considered as a useful, well-tolerated, but second-line and not very potent drug for Parkinson's disease. In the late 1980s amantadine reappeared in the literature as a drug that could improve motor fluctuations in patients on chronic levodopa therapy. This effect was modest and transient. Amantadine is a weak NMDA receptor antagonist that plugs the NMDA channel, preventing calcium entry into the nerve cell. It is well-tolerated in patients with Parkinson's disease and notably does not cause sedation.

Memantine is a structural analog of amantadine that is available in Europe for the treatment of Parkinson's disease. Like amantadine, it is considered to be a useful adjunct to levodopa therapy but not a first-line drug for Parkinson's disease. Memantine is a more potent blocker of the NMDA receptor channel than amantadine. Measurement of brain concentrations achieved with the recommended daily dose of memantine suggest that they are sufficient to antagonize NMDA receptors, yet this drug is not very sedating. The reason could be that memantine binds in a special way to the NMDA receptor channel, but it could also be that the drug plugs the channels associated only with certain subpopulations of NMDA receptors. Clinical trials with memantine are ongoing in the United States.

Although these older drugs may be helpful, there is clearly room for improvement, and the search for new NMDA antagonists is an active one. Most of these drugs are being tested for stroke, another condition that involves glutamate toxicity. The search for new channel blockers has been disappointing because most of them turned out to be toxic. Two inhibitors at the polyamine site, ifenprodil and eliprodil, have been discovered. They are not sedating and seem to induce few side effects. They are currently being tested in stroke patients but might also be useful for Parkinson's disease.

## ►CONCLUSION

There is rather strong evidence that an excess of free radicals is involved in Parkinson's disease. Decreasing the levels of these toxic chemicals in the substantia nigra could therefore slow the progression of Parkinson's disease.

This could be achieved with antioxidants that "mop up" free radicals or with drugs that decrease the production of free radicals in the substantia nigra, such as MAO-B inhibitors or glutamate antagonists. Drugs that block glutamate transmission could be beneficial in more than one way in Parkinson's disease. First, they could decrease and perhaps even eliminate peak-dose dyskinesias. Second, they may help slow the progression of the disease. Although it is unlikely that excess glutamate is the primary cause of Parkinson's disease, most investigators agree that glutamate, by increasing the energy demands on neurons, could make "sick" neurons even sicker.

# 14
# Neuronal Transplantation

Neural transplantation for the treatment of Parkinson's disease is not reported in the newspapers as often as it once was, but the field is very much alive, maturing and gaining in wisdom what it may have lost in early excitement. The hurdles that need to be overcome before neural transplantation is generally available remain impressive, but at least scientists have identified many of the difficulties.

The theory underlying neural transplantation is relatively simple. Since the loss of nerve cells in the substantia nigra causes the symptoms of the disease, replacing lost cells with new ones should reverse these symptoms. Many immediately obvious problems are associated with neural transplantation: What should be the source of nerve cells—fetal tissue or cell cultures? Will nerve cells survive after transplantation? Will the disease process that caused nerve cells to die in the first place also cause grafted nerve cells to die?

There are also less obvious issues:

- Nerve cells in the substantia nigra send projections (axons) to the nearby striatum, where their terminals liberate dopamine. The symptoms of Parkinson's disease are due to decreased levels of dopamine in the striatum. Grafted cells must therefore release dopamine in the striatum. At the present time, nerve cells placed in the substantia nigra do not send their axons to the striatum and release dopamine, and transplants are therefore placed directly into the striatum.

- Nerve cells in the substantia nigra normally receive inputs from several other brain areas. These connections are important for smooth motor function, but are lost when substantia nigra nerve cells die. Grafted cells would have to reestablish normal connections for completely normal motor function to occur. However, these connections are formed before birth, and we do not know how to make them happen in adults. Coaxing nerve cells from other brain regions to send axons back to the substantia nigra after they had withdrawn them will require a great deal of research.

Nerve cells transplanted into the striatum survive and continue to grow for at least several months. One patient with Parkinson's disease who had received bilateral fetal ventral mesencephalic grafts into a part of the striatum called the putamen showed some clinical improvement following surgery. Positron emission tomographic (PET) scans that could detect dopamine-producing neurons showed that the grafts were growing. When the patient died 18 months after transplantation, postmortem examination showed that the grafts had survived well and had grown an extensive network of neurites. This process takes time, which probably explains why patients show continued slow improvement for several years after transplantation.

This theory is supported by PET scans taken at regular intervals after surgery. Grafts survived for several years in all 13 patients in a study at the Lund University Hospital in Sweden. Two have now reached their sixth year post-surgery, and their grafts appear to be functioning well. When patients are grafted on only one side, PET scanning shows that the grafted cells survive and apparently do not decrease in number, while substantia nigra nerve cells continue to be lost on the other side. This proves that whatever process is causing nerve cells to die does not seem to affect the grafted cells.

Grafts not only survive for prolonged periods, but they also have beneficial effects. Symptom relief is still incomplete, but it does persist and improves slowly with time. One of the issues is therefore to obtain better relief of parkinsonian symptoms.

## ►ESTABLISHING NORMAL CONNECTIONS

Although the fact that grafts can survive is encouraging, the grafted nerve cells seem not to make good contacts with other cells. Specifically, nerve cells grafted in the substantia nigra do not send axons to the striatum. In people with Parkinson's disease, grafts are therefore placed directly into the striatum, where they make dopamine, grow short axons that make contact with the striatal nerve cells surrounding them, and liberate the neurotransmitter. The first objective of neural transplantation—to provide dopamine to the striatum—is fulfilled. However, these nerve cells grafted into the striatum do not receive the input that "normal" substantia nigra nerve cells receive from other brain regions (Figure 14.1). This incomplete connectivity may explain why grafted patients are only partially improved.

Research is therefore focused on how to encourage nerve cells to make proper connections. Investigators working on other brain regions have shown that axons from grafts placed at a distance from their normal region can find their targets in adult animals, suggesting that some regions of the brain still retain the anatomic cues that guide axonal growth over quite long distances. These results lead us to wonder why nerve cells grafted in the substantia nigra cannot make the relatively small one-inch "jump" to the striatum. Attempts are

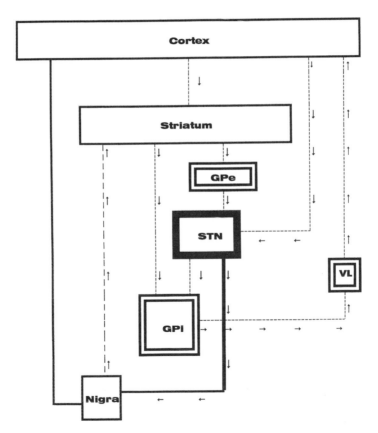

*Figure 14.1.* Schematic representation of efferent pathways from the striatum. In Parkinson's disease, neurons in the substantia nigra (nigra) die out. These neurons deliver dopamine to the striatum. Decreased levels of dopamine in the striatum are the cause of increased activity in the GPi (internal segment globus pallidum) and in the STN (subthalamic nucleus). VL: ventrolateral nucleus of thalamus; GPe: external segment globus pallidum.

being made to help grafted nerve cells send axons from the nigra to the striatum by implanting "guides" that bridge them. For example, fetal nerve cells grafted in the nigra can be guided to the striatum by an injury-induced factor. In this study, the axons released large amounts of dopamine in response to stimulation and were therefore functional.

## ►SOURCES OF NERVE CELLS FOR TRANSPLANTATION

Another problem with transplantation is obtaining nerve cells. Grafts currently are obtained from fetuses, which poses both ethical and practical problems. The difficulty in obtaining nerve cells is increased by the amount of tissue that is needed. Because 80–95 percent of grafted cells are lost immediately after transplantation, two to three fetuses are needed per grafted side. Minimizing nerve cell loss immediately after grafting would decrease this problem. The younger the donor cells, the better they survive. The age of the patient also affects survival—the younger the patient, the better the graft survives.

It is important to place the tissue in the appropriate area. Some regions of the brain are more "friendly" to grafts than others. Grafts also need to be rapidly vascularized (i.e., entered by blood vessels). The grafted cells survive and apparently do not decrease in number, which remains a problem. In animals adding a trophic factor such as beta-FGF (fibroblast growth factor) to a graft greatly increases the number of cells that survive, and injecting GDNF (glial cell line-derived neurotrophic factor) into the substantia nigra of parkinsonian monkeys significantly improved graft survival. The administration of free radical scavengers at the time of grafting has also proved helpful.

## ►IMMUNOSUPPRESSION AND GRAFTING

Grafting requires treatment with immunosuppressive agents to prevent graft rejection. This type of treatment can be dangerous but it is not required forever; several grafted patients have now been taken off immunosuppressant therapy and are doing well. We do not yet know how long immunosuppressant therapy should last.

Recently an elegant technique that provides localized immune suppression has been used in animals. It is based on a particular feature of Sertoli cells found in the testes, which protect sperm cells from immune attack. When these cells are injected together with nerve cells into the animal brain, they surround the nerve cells and protect them from being rejected by secreting immunosuppressant compounds. Sertoli cells also seem to secrete trophic factors that help the nerve cells grow and differentiate. This protective effect has been used for a number of other graft types; for example, Sertoli cells protect pancreatic cell grafts in diabetic animals.

## ▶TRANSPLANTATION OF DOPAMINE-PRODUCING CELLS

An alternative to neural transplantation would be to graft into the striatum cells that are genetically engineered to produce dopamine (see also the section in this chapter on genetic engineering). These cells are not nerve cells; rather they act like small dopamine factories placed directly into the striatum. They meet the first objective of transplantation, the delivery of dopamine to the striatum, but cannot establish normal connections with all the brain regions that usually "talk" to the substantia nigra neurons. The risk with these techniques therefore is that improvement will never be complete. In parkinsonian monkeys, grafts of cells genetically modified to make dopamine survived and showed improvement of symptoms.

Grafting genetically engineered cells that make dopamine into the striatum could have many advantages over taking levodopa. First, it would ensure a continuous and regular release of dopamine, affording a smooth antiparkinsonian effect without peak-dose side effects and end-of-dose loss of efficacy. Additionally, the continuous release of dopamine is probably desirable in Parkinson's disease to delay the onset of late-stage complications. The local delivery of dopamine directly into the striatum should have the added advantage of avoiding many of the side effects of levodopa therapy. The levels of dopamine would be very high in the immediate vicinity of the grafted cells and quite low in other areas of the striatum. This would be quite different from the "natural" situation in which dopamine levels are fairly constant throughout the striatum and might cause new types of side effects and problems.

Grafting genetically engineered cells could also help deliver neurotrophic factors to brain areas where nerve cells are dying. Because some neurotrophic factors protect nerve cells from death in animals, many investigators think that they might be beneficial in Parkinson's disease. Unfortunately, these factors are large proteins that are destroyed in the stomach when given by mouth and never reach the bloodstream; when injected intravenously, they do not enter the brain because of their size. Their delivery to the brain is therefore a major problem, which might be solved by using genetically engineered cells.

One biotechnology company has invented a system in which baby hamster kidney cells are modified to make nerve growth factor (NGF), which may be crucial in Alzheimer's disease. These cells are encapsulated within polymer membranes and implanted into the cerebral ventricles of rats. Encapsulation allows their removal completely and easily if needed. Thirteen months later, the capsules contained many healthy cells that were still making NGF. The same company recently showed that the technology can be used in humans. Cells developed to make a neurotrophic factor that may be helpful in ALS were encapsulated cells and placed close to the lesioned nerve cells in patients. Preliminary results showed that the grafts were well-tolerated. Thus, it may be possible to safely and efficiently deliver neurotrophic factors to brain regions where they are needed. The same group of scientists is also active in the field of Parkinson's disease and have engineered cells to make dopamine as well as cells to make glial cell line-derived neurotrophic factor (GDNF).

## ►TRANSPLANTATION OF STEM CELLS

Nerve cells are formed before birth from stem cells, as is shown in Figure 14.2. Until recently it was thought that no stem cells remained in the brain after birth because they had all differentiated into neurons or glia. Recent research has shown that a few, apparently quiescent, progenitor cells remain in the adult brain. These cells can be extracted and will survive indefinitely in the presence of a trophic factor, and so might be a readily available and practically unlimited source of nerve cells to graft. In animals progenitor cells injected into a lesioned part of the brain differentiate into glia rather than neurons that could replace those lost through disease. Progenitor cells injected into an *intact* part of the brain do become nerve cells; even more interestingly, they acquire the characteristics of striatal nerve cells if they are put into a healthy striatum and become hippocampal nerve cells if put into an area of the brain called the *hippocampus*. Current research involves studying various ways of injecting progenitor cells into lesioned substantia nigra in an attempt to force them to differentiate into nerve cells. This may take several years, and many technical difficulties will probably need to be overcome. Another research goal is to find factors that would "coax" the

**Stem Cells → Progenitor Cells**  ↗ **Nerve Cells**  ↘ **Glial Cells**

Figure 14.2. Schematic representation of nerve cell differentiation. Stem cells, progenitor cells, and glial cells can multiply; nerve cells cannot.

few remaining stem cells in the substantia nigra to differentiate and replace lost nerve cells.

# ▶GENETIC ENGINEERING

The technology of genetic engineering could be used two ways in Parkinson's disease.

- It could be used to design cells that will produce specific substances, such as dopamine, that can be transplanted into the appropriate brain region, a technology called *in vitro* gene therapy.
- Genes could be directly introduced into specific cells, such as those of the substantia nigra. Such *in vivo* gene therapy is at a very early stage of research. Enormous difficulties must be overcome before patients can benefit from such techniques, and it may never be possible to safely give people new genetic material instead of medication.

Many technical hurdles must be overcome before grafts of genetically engineered cells can be made available to patients. For example:

- Grafted cells must survive in their new environment. Parkinsonian (MPTP) monkeys have been extremely useful in finding out what factors influence cell survival.
- Grafted cells must make the correct amount of the desired substance, neither too much nor too little.
- There must be a way to turn off production: this is now possible by coupling the inserted gene to a switch that responds to drugs like antibiotics; the gene stops production if the patient stops taking the drug.
- There must be a way to remove the grafted cells if needed: one way to do this would be to insert an additional gene in the cells (a "death" gene), which is turned on by a specific drug. If the grafted cells needed to be removed, the patient would be given this drug and the grafted cells would die.

Another interesting application of genetic engineering to the treatment of Parkinson's disease would be to use cells engineered to make levodopa rather than dopamine. They would be implanted under the skin to become a stable and continuous source of levodopa. This technique is similar to intravenous infusion and would overcome the problems linked to fluctuating levels of levodopa in the bloodstream. However, patients would need to take an oral decarboxylase inhibitor to prevent the formation of dopamine in the bloodstream (see Chapter 2) and the development of unpleasant side effects, such as vomiting and decreased blood pressure.

## ▶GENES TO TREAT PARKINSON'S DISEASE

Another way to cause certain proteins to be made in the brain would be to inject into patients the genes that make a protein, with the hope that the injected gene will cause cells to make it. For this to happen, the injected gene must both enter the right cells and be incorporated into their chromosomes. This could be done in several ways. Even when the gene has been successfully incorporated into the right cell, all would not necessarily be well. The new gene would have to go to the right place in the chromosome, or at least not to a place where it might cause a disease such as cancer. It must make the right protein (sometimes when genes become part of a chromosome, they make proteins different from the ones they are supposed to code for), and it must make them in the right amounts. Ideally, the new gene should go only to the cells where the protein needs to be made, but how can a gene know which cells to colonize? The technical hurdles that need to be overcome are impressive, and it will probably be many years before this type of therapy can be offered to people with Parkinson's disease.

Various methods can be used to introduce genes into cells. For example, a gene can be inserted into an inactivated virus (that will not cause brain disease) that preferentially colonizes nerve cells. Herpes simplex is particularly well suited for this because it has a strong preference for nerve cells, can be reliably inactivated, contains many nonessential genes that can be removed to make space for the new genes, and expresses inserted genes in a stable and predictable manner. One of the many issues involved in this type of treatment will be to find ways to colonize specific nerve cells. In the case of Parkinson's disease, for example, it is possible to insert into herpes simplex a gene that is critical for making dopamine. This gene, however, should only be expressed in the substantia nigra or in the striatum, and herpes simplex does not seem to distinguish between nerve cells.

Stem cells can be isolated from the brain and made to express a particular gene when they are injected back into the brain; they can therefore be used to deliver genes to the brain.

Another approach, *biolistic gene transfer*, involves coating microscopic gold particles with genes, introducing a needle into the brain region where they are needed, and "shooting" the coated particles through the needle under high pressure. Under these conditions brain cells are not lesioned and a significant number of them incorporate the new genes. This technique has been used for several years to introduce genes into plants, but it is just beginning to be studied for the brain and has at the present time only been used in animals. It has several advantages, and is safe, fast, easy, and inexpensive. One of the problems will be to obtain prolonged expression of the injected genes. At present, expression lasts for only a few days.

## CONCLUSION

At the present time, brain transplants provide only modest improvement, and research is actively ongoing to solve some of the major problems linked to this procedure. The use of genetically engineered cells would be somewhat similar to brain transplants, but it is still at a very early stage of development. Most investigators agree that it will take at least 15 years before transplantation becomes a reliable treatment for Parkinson's disease.

# *Appendix A*

## GLOSSARY

**Acetylcholine**   Neurotransmitter involved in many brain functions, notably memory and the control of motor activity.

**Alpha-tocopherol**   Chemical name for vitamin E.

**Alzheimer's disease**   A neurodegenerative disorder in which several neuronal systems degenerate, including a group of cholinergic neurons located at the base of the brain.

**Amantadine (Symmetrel®)**   Sometimes used as initial therapy of Parkinson's disease, it may slow disease progression. Its mechanism of action is unclear; some think it exerts its beneficial effects by blocking NMDA receptors.

**Amyotrophic lateral sclerosis**   A neurodegenerative disorder also known as Lou Gehrig's disease. The gene responsible for the familial form has been identified and codes for a protein involved in free radical scavenging.

**Apomorphine**   Oldest known dopamine agonist. It is not active by mouth, but works almost as well as levodopa when it is infused intravenously.

**Apoptosis**   A form of cell death in which cells shrink and disappear. It is sometimes referred to as "cell suicide" and was first described more than 40 years ago. Many think that in Parkinson's disease substantia nigra nerve cells die by apoptosis.

**Artane®**   Anticholinergic drug used for the treatment of Parkinson's disease.

**Atypical parkinsonism**   Also referred to as parkinson plus, this is a group of many diseases that may, at onset, look like Parkinson's disease, but differ from it by their brain lesions, clinical features, clinical course, and response to antiparkinsonian medications. Because the majority of these "look-alike" illnesses are due to the loss of more than one set of neurons, they are also called multiple systems atrophy.

**Autonomic nervous system dysfunction**   A group of symptoms that includes problems with blood pressure, sweating, and sexual function.

**bcl-2 gene**   Gene that prevents apoptosis in human cells.

**BDNF (brain-derived-neurotrophic factor)**   Neurotrophic factor for substantia nigra nerve cells that seems to act mainly at the early stages of development.

**Benign essential tremor**    A common condition that is often familial and affects up to three million Americans. It is sometimes mistaken for Parkinson's disease, but there is no stiffness or slowness.

**Benserazide**    Inhibitor of an enzyme called decarboxylase; it does not penetrate well into the brain, and therefore inhibits the enzyme mainly outside the brain.

**Bradykinesia**    Slowness of bodily movements (from the Greek, *brady* meaning slow, and *kinesia* meaning movement); it is one of the three symptoms of the triad that characterizes Parkinson's disease.

**Bromocriptine (Parlodel®)**    Dopamine agonist used for the treatment of Parkinson's disease; it stimulates mainly the D2 dopamine receptor.

**Cabergoline**    Dopamine agonist that stimulates mainly the D2 dopamine receptor. It has a long half-life, is commercially available and is used for the treatment of Parkinson's disease in Europe, but not yet in the United States.

***Caenorhabditis elegans (C. elegans):*** A microscopic worm in which the genes that control apoptosis as well as the genes that influence aging have been studied. Scientists use this worm because it is a relatively easy model system with which to work.

**Carbidopa**    Inhibitor of an enzyme called decarboxylase; like benserazide, it does not penetrate well into the brain, and therefore inhibits the enzyme mainly outside the brain.

**Catechol-ortho-methyl transferase (COMT)**    Enzyme that converts levodopa to 3-O-methyldopa.

**Chromosomes**    Long chains of genes. Most cells in our body have a nucleus that contains chromosomes arranged by pairs. Human beings have 23 pairs of chromosomes; within each pair of chromosomes, one comes from the father and one comes from the mother.

**Cisapride**    Drug that accelerates gastric emptying and intestinal transit; it can be beneficial in patients with Parkinson's disease.

**Clinical trial**    A scientific study conducted in patients to evaluate whether a new treatment is beneficial and safe.

**Clinical trial protocol**    Written plan of the procedures that will be done during a clinical trial; it must be approved by the Institutional Review Board before the trial starts.

**Clock genes**    Genes involved in the aging process.

**Clozapine**    Drug used for the treatment of psychiatric diseases; it blocks mainly the D4 dopamine receptor and may help alleviate mental symptoms caused by levodopa without worsening motor symptoms of Parkinson's disease.

**Cogentin®**    Anticholinergic drug used for the treatment of Parkinson's disease.

**Complex-1**    Part of the mitochondria, which is often damaged in Parkinson's disease.

**COMT inhibitors**    Compounds that increase the half-life of levodopa by preventing its degradation by COMT.

**Corpus striatum**    Anatomical term referring to a brain region that plays an essential role in motor activity. In Parkinson's disease the concentrations of dopamine in the corpus striatum are profoundly reduced, causing the motor symptoms of the disease.

**CPP-32**    Enzyme that promotes apoptosis in human cells.

**Cytochrome P450 system**    A special group of enzymes in the liver that transform (i.e., metabolize) substances we ingest, including medications; it has been suggested that this system is abnormal in Parkinson's disease.

**Cytokines**    Proteins made by immune cells as well as many other cells. They act as powerful messengers from one cell to another, and the messages they carry deal with cell growth, survival, or death.

**Decarboxylase (DC)**    Enzyme that converts levodopa to dopamine.

**Depression**    A disorder that is often associated with Parkinson's disease and involves many symptoms such as sadness, loss of pleasure in most activities, irritability, loss of energy, poor appetite, and insomnia.

**Dextromethorphan}**    Active ingredient of cough syrups; in high doses it blocks NMDA receptors.

**Dihedrexidine**    A new drug that stimulates D1 dopamine receptors.

**Domperidone**    Drug that blocks dopamine D2 receptors; it does not penetrate well into the striatum. It is used to prevent nausea and vomiting in patients with Parkinson's disease. It is commercially available in Europe and Canada but not in the United States.

**Dopa (3,4-dihydroxyphenylalanine)**    A substance found in plants and in animals. It exists in two forms: the L- and the D-forms; only the L-form (called levodopa) exists in nature.

**Dopamine**    Chemical substance made by certain nerve cells, notably substantia nigra nerve cells. It is a neurotransmitter whose concentrations in the striatum are profoundly decreased in Parkinson's disease.

**Dopamine agonists**    Substances that stimulate dopamine receptors and mimic the effects of dopamine. They are used for the treatment of Parkinson's disease.

**Dopamine antagonists**    Substances that block dopamine receptors and prevent the effects of dopamine. They are used for the treatment of psychiatric disorders, as well as for the treatment of nausea and other gastrointestinal complaints. They sometimes cause parkinsonism.

**Dopamine receptors**    Proteins located on the surface of certain nerve cells, they selectively recognize and bind dopamine. There are four known dopamine receptors, called D1, D2, D3, and D4.

**Double-blind clinical trial**    A trial in which neither the patient nor the physician knows what treatment the patient is receiving. Conducting a trial double-blind prevents bias. Health authorities (i.e., Food and Drug Administration in the United States) require that a drug's benefits be demonstrated in double-blind studies before it is commercialized.

**Dyskinesia**    Abnormal involuntary movement.

**Dystonia**    Painful sustained muscle contraction.

**Eliprodil**    A new drug that blocks the glycine site of the NMDA receptor.

**Encephalitis**    A brain inflammation usually caused by a virus (from the Greek *encephalon,* meaning brain, and *-itis,* meaning inflammation).

**Entalcapone**    A new drug that blocks COMT and therefore prolongs the effects of levodopa.

**Free radicals**    Toxic substances that are continuously produced by all cells of the human body; their concentrations are particularly high in the substantia nigra. They may be involved in the loss of nerve cells that characterizes Parkinson's disease.

**Free radical scavenging systems**    Free radicals are normally "scavenged" by a complicated system of enzymes (antioxidant enzymes) and vitamins such as vitamin E and vitamin C. The action of antioxidants on free radicals is comparable to that of a sponge on water. Antioxidants "mop up" free radicals.

**Freezing**    A feature of the parkinsonian gait disorder. Patients who are walking well suddenly find their feet and legs completely immobilized or "frozen" to the ground for a few seconds.

**GDNF (glial-cell-line-derived neurotrophic factor)**    Neurotrophic factor liberated by glial cells and that acts on substantia nigra nerve cells. Unlike BDNF, which seems to act primarily on young nerve cells, GDNF may play a major role in the survival of adult substantia nigra neurons.

**Genes**    Long sequences of DNA; they are the basis of heredity and are like the blueprint for the proteins in our body. They can be "switched" on or off. When a gene is "switched on," the protein it codes for is produced. Familial diseases often involve an abnormal gene.

**Gene therapy**    Use of genes to treat human diseases. The challenge is to get specific genes into the cells that need them and to make the genes function in the new cell. Several methods of gene delivery are being investigated.

**Genetic engineering**    Technology used to force cells or bacteria to make certain proteins. Genes are "clipped out" of a chromosome and "inserted" into the chromosome of another cell. In other words, genetic engineering consists of "cutting and pasting" genes. This type of technology is used to prepare cells for transplantation. It also enables scientists to obtain large amounts of proteins that are difficult to make.

**Globus pallidum**   Anatomical structure of the brain involved in motor function; it is the target of pallidotomy.

**Glutamate**   Neurotransmitter involved in many brain functions; in high concentrations it can kill nerve cells.

**High frequency electrical stimulation**   Also referred to as deep brain stimulation, it is a surgical technique that paralyzes small groups of nerve cells by subjecting them to high frequency electrical currents through electrodes implanted in the brain.

**Huntington's disease**   An inherited neurodegenerative disorder characterized by the progressive loss of a group of neurons located in the corpus striatum. The gene for the disease was recently identified; it may be involved in the pathways that lead to apoptosis.

**Immune system**   Network of several different types of cells and organs that work together to defend the body against invasion by foreign substances.

**Immunosuppression**   Treatment to prevent graft and transplant rejection.

**Informed consent**   Subject's consent to participate in a clinical trial after the risks and potential benefits have been fully explained.

**Institutional Review Board (IRB)**   A committee made up of scientists, doctors, clergy, and other people from the community, whose function is to protect patients who participate in clinical trials.

**Interferons**   Family of cytokines; there are at least three types of interferons (interferon-alpha, interferon-beta, and interferon-gamma).

**Interleukin-1-beta**   A cytokine made by many cells of the body, including brain cells. It is a powerful promoter of apoptosis.

**Interleukin-1-beta converting enzyme (ICE)**   Enzyme that converts the inactive precursor of interleukin-1-beta to the active cytokine.

**Iron chelators**   Substances that bind to iron and eliminate it from the body.

**Lazabemide**   A new drug that inhibits type B monoamine oxidase and could therefore be beneficial in Parkinson's disease.

**Levodopa**   Natural substance found in a number of plants. It is the precursor to dopamine and is currently the best treatment for Parkinson's disease; it is the active ingredient of Sinemet® and Madopar®.

**Lewy bodies**   Pink iridescent spheres found in dying substantia nigra nerve cells. These inclusions are the hallmark of Parkinson's disease.

**Livido reticularis**   Purplish or bluish mottling of the skin caused by certain antiparkinsonian treatments such as amantadine.

**Lou Gehrig's disease**   A neurodegenerative disorder also called amyotrophic lateral sclerosis.

**Madopar®**   A combination of levodopa and benserazide that is used as a treatment for Parkinson's disease.

**Madopar HBS®**   A special formulation that contains Madopar®. HBS stands for hydrodynamically balanced system. Madopar HBS® releases levodopa slowly in the stomach.

**Memantine**   A new drug that is a powerful analog of amantadine and blocks the NMDA receptor.

**Microglia**   Cells of the immune system that are found exclusively in the brain; they are thought to be a subset of phagocytes.

**Micrographia**   Small handwriting often observed in people with Parkinson's disease.

**Mitochondria**   Small cigar-shaped organelles present in all cells. Their role is to provide energy to cells. They are also the "lungs" of the cell; they "breathe in" oxygen and "breathe out" free radicals.

**Monoamine oxidase (MAO)**   Enzyme that degrades several substances in the brain, including dopamine. There are two types of MAOs, type A and type B. The latter degrades dopamine in the brain; this reaction involves the formation of toxic free radicals.

**Monoamine oxidase inhibitors**   Drugs that block MAO. Type B inhibitors prolong the duration of action of dopamine; they may also slow the progression of Parkinson's disease (*see also* Selegiline).

**MPP+**   Toxic substance formed from MPTP; it paralyzes Complex-1 in the mitochondria.

**MPTP**   Toxic substance that destroys substantia nigra neurons and causes parkinsonism in humans, monkeys, and other animal species.

**Multiple systems atrophy**   Group of neurodegenerative disorders that share some common features with Parkinson's disease but differ on a number of points (*see* Atypical parkinsonism).

**Necrosis**   A form of cell death in which cells swell, explode, and die.

**Neurodegenerative disorders**   Group of illnesses that affect the brain and spinal cord and include conditions such as Parkinson's disease, Alzheimer's disease, Huntington's disease, amyotrophic lateral sclerosis (ALS, or Lou Gehrig's disease). Neurodegenerative disorders are characterized by the gradual loss of certain sets of nerve cells in specific areas of the brain.

**Neuroleptics**   Drugs that block dopamine receptors; they belong to the group of dopamine antagonists and are used to treat psychiatric disorders.

**Neuromelanin**   Substance made by substantia nigra neurons; its production involves the liberation of free radicals.

**Neurotransmitters**   Chemical substances that carry messages from one nerve cell to an other. Dopamine is a neurotransmitter.

**Neurotrophic factors** Substances that prevent nerve cells from committing apoptosis.

**NMDA receptor** One of glutamate's receptors (glutamate is a neurotransmitter).

**Olivopontocerebellar atrophy (OPCA)** A multiple system atrophy; the term *OPCA* covers a heterogeneous group of neurodegenerative conditions with loss of nerve cells in the pons, cerebellum, and often substantia nigra and spinal cord.

**On-off effect** A symptom usually observed in late stages of Parkinson's disease, it is characterized by rapid fluctuations from a state of parkinsonism to a normal state.

**OPC-14117** Experimental drug that scavenges free radicals in the brain.

**Orthostatic hypotension** Sudden and profound decreases in blood pressure when changing from lying to standing or from sitting to standing position; it can cause fainting.

**Pallidotomy** Stereotactic surgical procedure that destroys cells in a brain region called globus pallidum and improves some symptoms of Parkinson's disease.

**Parkinson plus** A group of diseases also referred to as "atypical parkinsonism."

**Parkinson's disease** Slowly progressive neurodegenerative disorder first described by James Parkinson in 1817. The disease is characterized by the association of tremor, bradykinesia, and rigidity. These symptoms are due to the gradual loss of nerve cells in a small brain region called the substantia nigra.

**Parkinsonian triad** The three cardinal symptoms of Parkinson's disease: tremor, bradykinesia, and rigidity.

**Parkinsonism** Group of symptoms including tremor, rigidity, bradykinesia, stooped posture, and shuffling gait. Parkinsonism is most often the consequence of Parkinson's disease; it can sometimes be caused by drugs that block the dopamine D2 receptor, in which case it is usually reversible.

**Pergolide (Permax®)** Dopamine agonist that stimulates mainly the D2 dopamine receptor; it is used for the treatment of Parkinson's disease.

**PET (positron emission tomography)** Imaging method that allows one to visualize brain dopamine systems following the injection of a radioactive analog of levodopa (fluorodopa).

**p53 gene** Gene that causes apoptosis in human cells, possibly by switching off the bcl-2 gene.

**Phagocytes** Cells of the immune system that patrol for foreign substances and give the alarm when they find foreign or abnormal cells.

**Pramipexole** A new drug that stimulates D2 and D3 dopamine receptors.

**Progressive supranuclear palsy (PSP)** The most common of the "atypical parkinsonism" disorders; it is often confused with Parkinson's disease during its initial course.

**Prolactin**   Hormone that controls lactation. D2 dopamine receptor agonists decrease its blood levels.

**Randomization**   Procedure used in clinical trials to avoid bias. Patients are allocated to one or the other treatment by chance.

**Retrocollis**   Tendency for the neck to bend back and up.

**Rigidity**   Muscle stiffness; it is one of the three symptoms of the parkinsonian triad.

**Ropinirole**   A new drug that stimulates mainly dopamine D2 receptors.

**Selegiline**   MAO inhibitor that blocks mainly type B MAO; given to patients with early Parkinson's disease, it may delay the need for levodopa.

**Sertoli cells**   Found in the testes, these cells secrete immunosuppressant substances that ensure local protection against graft rejection.

**Shaking palsy**   Term used by James Parkinson to describe Parkinson's disease.

**Shy-Drager syndrome**   A multiple systems atrophy; the disease is characterized by autonomic insufficiency combined with parkinsonian and cerebellar features.

**Sinemet®**   A combination of levodopa and carbidopa used as a treatment for Parkinson's disease.

**Sinemet CR®**   Tablet of Sinemet® encased in a special matrix; it dissolves slowly in the stomach and in the bowel, allowing for a prolonged, steady absorption of levodopa into the bloodstream.

**Six-hydroxydopamine**   Toxic substance that destroys substantia nigra nerve cells

**Sleep apnea**   Disorder characterized by frequent pauses in breathing that happen only during sleep.

**Spinocerebellar atrophy**   *See* Olivopontocerebellar atrophy.

**Stereotactic surgery**   Surgical technique that allows the destruction of small brain regions without directly visualizing the area to be ablated.

**Striatonigral degeneration**   A disease that belongs to the group of atypical parkinsonism.

**Striatum**   Short for corpus striatum.

**Substantia nigra**   Anatomical term referring to a brain region located deep in the brainstem. There is a left and a right substantia nigra. In Parkinson's disease the nerve cells in the substantia nigra die, and this causes the motor symptoms of the disease.

**Superoxidedismutase (SOD)**   Enzyme that scavenges free radicals; it is abnormal in the familial forms of amyotrophic lateral sclerosis.

**Tolcapone**   A new drug that inhibits COMT and therefore prolongs the effects of levodopa.

**Tremor**  Often the first symptom of Parkinson's disease, it is one of the three symptoms of the parkinsonian triad.

**Tumor-necrosing-factor-alpha (TNF-alpha)**  A cytokine that is a powerful promoter of apoptosis for most cells. In the brain, however, it may oppose apoptosis. Its levels are increased in the substantia nigra of people with Parkinson's disease.

**Vitamin E**  A vitamin that protects cells from free radical damage; it does not seem to be helpful in Parkinson's disease, perhaps because it does not penetrate well into the brain.

**Vomiting center**  Anatomical term describing a group of cells in a brain region called medulla oblongata. These cells initiate and coordinate the act of vomiting. They are very sensitive to drugs that stimulate dopamine transmission.

**von Economo's encephalitis**  Named after the Austrian neurologist who first described the condition, it is a form of encephalitis that causes progressive parkinsonism.

**Wearing-off**  Also referred to as end-of-dose deterioration; it is a late-stage motor complication characterized by the progressive shortening of the effect of each dose of levodopa.

# Appendix B

## RESOURCES

### Patient Voluntary Organizations

In the United States there are several nonprofit voluntary organizations that provide patient service and research support in the field of Parkinson's disease. The major voluntary agencies in the United States working on Parkinson's disease are:

- The American Parkinson Disease Association, Inc.
  1250 Hylan Boulevard
  Staten Island, NY 10305
  Tel: (718) 981-8001; (800) 223-2732; fax: (718) 981-4300)

- The National Parkinson Foundation, Inc.
  1501 Ninth Avenue/Bob Hope Road
  Miami, FL 33136
  Tel: (305) 547-6666; information lines: (800) 327-4545;
  in Florida (800) 433-7022; in California: (800) 400-8448

- The Parkinson's Disease Foundation
  William Black Medical Research Building
  650-710 West 168th Street
  New York, NY 10032
  Tel: (212) 923-4700; (800) 457-6676; fax: (212) 92-4778

- United Parkinson Foundation
  833 West Washington Boulevard
  Chicago, IL 60607
  Tel: (312) 733-1893

The American Parkinson Disease Association (APDA) was founded in the early 1960s and grew rapidly to a national organization. It supports a national program of patient service including clinics and information centers throughout the United States. Local chapters organize patient education symposia featuring presentations by leading investigators in the field of

Parkinson's disease. The association also publishes a quarterly newsletter, booklets, and other informational materials. In addition to its efforts in the field of patient education, the APDA also sponsors basic and clinical research programs conducted at academic institutions throughout the country. It does this by awarding two and three year research grants and by sponsoring the George Cotzias fellowship, which provides research support and stipends to young scientists for three years, provided they conduct research in the field of Parkinson's disease.

The National Parkinson Foundation (NPF) was established in 1957. Its early efforts were mainly devoted to operating an outpatient clinic in Miami, Florida. Later the NPF began to award research grants to investigators throughout the United States. In 1986 it started a third line of activities consisting of identifying and supporting centers of excellence for Parkinson's disease research in the United States, Europe, and Japan. More than 40 such centers are currently in operation. The NPF sponsors international symposia on Parkinson's disease and publishes the proceedings. It also publishes a quarterly newsletter for patients and their families and several informational pamphlets.

The Parkinson's Disease Foundation was established in 1957 to support research into the cause of Parkinson's disease with the hope of eventually finding a cure. The foundation sponsors a broad basic and clinical research program on Parkinson's disease at the Columbia Presbyterian Medical Center in New York City. It also publishes a newsletter and organizes symposia for physicians and caregivers.

The United Parkinson Foundation (UPF) was founded in Chicago in 1963 to provide patients and their families with the knowledge needed to understand Parkinson's disease. The UPF devotes much of its activities to patient services, but it also funds grants to support research in Parkinson's disease.

Voluntary agencies have also been developed in Canada, in most European countries, and in Japan. Most of them are members of the International Federation of Parkinson Societies.

The Parkinson Foundation of Canada, Suite 232, ManuLife Center, 55 Bloor Street West, Toronto, Ontario, Canada M4W 1A6, was founded in the 1960s to provide service to patients and to support research. It operates through a network of local chapters and self-help groups to help patients and their families. The foundation also funds several research grants to scientists working on Parkinson's disease in Canada.

The Parkinson Disease Society of the United Kingdom, 36 Portland Place, London W1N 3DG, UK (tel: 071-255-2432) was formed in 1969 with the goal of helping patients and their families cope with Parkinson's disease. The society has grown to over 200 branches throughout the United Kingdom. One of its major contributions to Parkinson's disease research is the maintenance of a brain bank in London.

## WHERE TO OBTAIN INFORMATION ABOUT ONGOING CLINICAL TRIALS IN PARKINSON'S DISEASE

Unlike what exists for other diseases such as AIDS and cancer, there is no computerized, on-line listing of ongoing clinical trials in Parkinson's disease. Information on some of the trials can be obtained from the National Institute of Neurological Disorders and Stroke (NINDS) or from the Parkinson Study Group (PSG).

The NINDS in Bethesda, Maryland, is one of the National Institutes of Health (NIH). It conducts research on Parkinson's disease in its own research laboratories and maintains an active program of clinical research at the clinical center, a large hospital located in Bethesda. In the 1970s the NINDS established the Experimental Therapeutics Branch (ETB), which actively searches for new treatments for Parkinson's disease and tests new drugs in animals and in patients. Information concerning clinical trials conducted at ETB can be obtained from the ETB at (301) 496-6609. Patients who are interested in participating in clinical trials will usually be asked to have their physician send or fax a letter of referral and a case summary to Dr. Thomas Chase, Experimental Therapeutics Branch, NINDS/NIH, Building 10, Room 5C106, Bethesda, Maryland 20892-1406.

The Parkinson Study Group (PSG) is a consortium of 38 physicians in the United States and Canada, devoted to conducting multicenter clinical trials in Parkinson's disease. This is the group that conducted the now famous DATATOP study to examine whether selegiline (Deprenyl®) could slow the progression of Parkinson's disease. The results of this study were published in 1989. As a consequence, many researchers were convinced that it was possible to show that a drug slows or stops disease progression in patients, thus providing major impetus to the pharmaceutical industry to look for cures for the disease. The PSG continues to study the effects of new drugs in patients with Parkinson's disease. Information about ongoing clinical trials can be obtained by calling the PSG Coordination Center in Rochester, New York, at (716) 275-7311.

## HOME PHARMACY FOR PATIENTS WITH PARKINSON'S DISEASE

Athena Rx Home Pharmacy works closely with a number of national Parkinson's disease organizations to provide patients with products and services specific to their needs. Some of the benefits provided by Athena Rx include free express delivery of prescription orders, refill reminder notices, emergency pharmacists consultation on a 24-hour basis, and a subscription to the newsletter "Neurology Awareness." Athena Rx also provides customers with access to a variety of other resources designed for those with a neurologic condition, such as exercise video programs and self-help books on a number of different topics to assist in the day-to-day management of the condition. They can be reached toll-free at 1-800-5 ATHENA (1-800-528-4362).

## WHERE TO FIND INFORMATION ON RESEARCH IN PARKINSON'S DISEASE

At the beginning of each calendar year the NINDS makes available an annual summary of research on Parkinson's disease. Copies can be obtained by writing to the Office of Scientific and Health Reports, NINDS, Building 31, Room 8A16, National Institutes of Health, Bethesda MD 20892; tel: (301) 496-5751.

The Parkinson's Web (http://neuro-chief-e.mgh.harvard.edu/parkinsons web/Main/PDmain.html.) is an international nonprofit effort to use the Internet as an on-line archive of information on Parkinson's disease, its treatment, strategies for coping, and research news. It is intended for patients, their families, and friends. Further information can be obtained from Ken Bernstein, President of the Young Parkinson's Chapter of Massachusetts and coordinator of the Parkinson's Web; tel: (617) 527-2803; fax (617) 527-2077; or email cocosolo@aol.com.

"Parkinson's Disease Update" is a monthly newsletter devoted to bringing information on the most current medical, social, and psychological aspects of Parkinson's disease. Its publisher, Leon Charles Sack, has Parkinson's disease and firmly believes in the value of disseminating research news on the disease as quickly as possible, to bring relief to all those who suffer from the disease and also to help find a cure. More information can be obtained from the Medical Publishing Company, P.O. Box 450, Huntingdon Valley, PA 19006; tel: (215) 947-6648; fax: (215) 947-2552.

# Index